SLIPS, TRIPS AND FRACTURED HIPS

The ultimate guide to accident prevention and first aid; helping us stay safe, healthy and active as we get older.

Emma Hammett

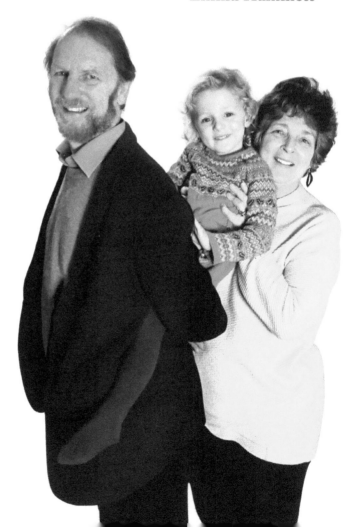

Published by First Aid for Life

Slips, Trips and Fractured Hips has been written by Emma Hammett, qualified nurse, first aid trainer and founder of First Aid for Life and onlinefirstaid.com in conjunction with other medical, first aid, health and emergency services professionals.

The contents are based on the Resuscitation Council UK guidance, European Research Council guidance on First Aid (ERC) and ILCOR (International Liaison Committee on Resuscitation) recommendations. The information is current at the time of publication and will be reviewed and updated with new editions.

Disclaimer: the author has made every effort to ensure the accuracy of the information contained within this book and whilst the book offers guidance it does not replace medical help. The author does not accept any liability or responsibility for any inaccuracies or for any mistreatment or misdiagnosis of any person or animal, however caused. If you suspect illness or injury, you should always seek immediate professional medical advice.

Slips, Trips and Fractured Hips

The ultimate guide to accident prevention and first aid; helping us stay safe, healthy and active as we get older.

Slips, Trips and Fractured Hips has been written for people caring for older friends and relatives; children caring for parents, for spouses, for older people wanting to keep themselves that bit safer and for anyone working with or caring for older people. It is designed to help you take measures to prevent life-threatening injuries and help you plan, prepare and avoid mishap. The aim is to enable people to remain safe, healthy and independent. *Slips, Trips and Fractured Hips* will equip you with the necessary skills should an accident occur. Immediate and appropriate first aid saves lives, reduces pain and suffering and can make a dramatic difference to the speed and extent of the casualty's recovery.

I am a qualified nurse and first aid trainer and have well over 30 years' experience in healthcare and first aid. In these roles, I have seen time and again how important prompt and appropriate first aid is in those crucial first few minutes following an accident. Yet so many people still lack the vital skills needed to make a difference when it matters most.

I am an acknowledged expert on first aid and accident prevention and frequently appear in the press and on TV. I have regular expert columns in various publications including The British Journal of School Nursing and the Journal of Family Health. I established First Aid for Life in 2007 and it has grown steadily to become a multi award-winning practical and online first aid training business. Our training has equipped thousands of carers, parents, teenagers, sports/health professionals and caring members of the public with the skills and confidence to help in a medical emergency. My motivation for founding First Aid for Life came from the numerous patients I saw who could have benefited from first aid. When working in medicine for the elderly, I saw numerous patients admitted for whom basic first aid would have made such a difference to their recovery. Elderly people are particularly vulnerable to shock (even though they may not show symptoms), ulcerating wounds and hypothermia. They may appear fine at first but without the right care will deteriorate extremely quickly. They can also experience quite major injury with surprisingly little force. I remember one diabetic patient in particular who had no idea of the amount of damage that had been done when they stubbed their toe and they ended up losing their foot as a result.

First aid treatment can be so simple, and knowing what to do can save people so much pain, scarring and further major hospital intervention.

As a mother, daughter and member of a huge, close family, I continually use my first aid knowledge and am forever grateful that I have the skill to quickly judge how seriously hurt or ill someone is and know the best way to help. This has enabled me to calmly administer first aid to my family at home and saved countless unnecessary trips to hospital.

Slips, Trips and Fractured Hips is packed full of practical hints and tips relevant to people as they get older.

The content of this book is supported by our practical first aid training (www.firstaidforlife.org.uk) and our online courses (www.onlinefirstaid. com), both of which help to make first aid skills more accessible to everyone. There are lots of helpful free resources and courses available on both these sites.

Forewords

"This useful little book, Slips, Trips and Fractured Hips is a bible of good sense and will encourage and advise you in ways to keep safe, healthy, actively upright and chirpy and reminds us that all is not lost with ageing and wonderful times can still lie ahead.

Preventing accidents from happening in the first place is, of course, the best option but when there are problems this excellent book is packed full of practical and sound advice.

It is there to help you enjoy your life to hilt. Please use it"

Carolyn Cripps OBE - Fit for Safety UK, Executive Committees of the Institute of Home Safety; the London Home and Water Safety Council, RoSPA's National Home Safety Committee and Trustee of Lambeth Age UK

"Falls and fragility fractures can result in loss of independence, injury and death. In health service terms, they are high volume and costly. A&E departments treat a disproportionate number of unintentional injuries among older people, and particularly those aged over 70, with accidents in the home (predominantly falls) accounting for the greatest proportion of these injuries.

In Slips, Trips and Fractured Hips, Emma discusses safety in relation to older people and uses her many years of experience to give good advice about preventing the most common accidents. Falls and other unintentional injuries are not an inevitable part of ageing and we hope that through the advice given in this book, older people and their loved ones will be able to take steps to prevent them from happening"

Sheila Merrill FRSPH UKPH - Public Health Adviser at The Royal Society for the Prevention of Accidents (RoSPA)

Introduction

As we get older our physiology changes and we often develop additional medical conditions. These conditions and the medicine taken to manage them can alter the way our bodies react to injury. Understanding this is key to managing a first aid emergency in an older person and anticipating how they might react to the injuries you can see. Staying one step ahead in an emergency situation often proves vital to the recovery of the casualty.

As we age, we also become more accident prone. Our eyesight deteriorates, our skin becomes more friable, we may develop medical conditions which affect our balance and mobility and generally we become more susceptible to injury. It is vital that we recognise this and take extra steps to keep ourselves fit and healthy and are mindful of common avoidable hazards that frequently lead to accidental injury.

More than 4,500 people in England over the age of 65 were recorded as having died as a result of a fall in 2015 (RoSPA).

This is likely to be the tip of the iceberg as falls, although not necessarily the cause of death, can result in a significant decline in health, contributing to many more deaths than this figure implies.

Older people can suffer serious injuries from falls, bleeds and burns that would be superficial in a younger person. They may not respond to a medical emergency in the usual way and can deteriorate extremely quickly. It is important to recognise and understand that the physiology in older people is different and that medication may affect this too. *Slips, Trips and Fractured Hips*

- Has a fit for the first time, even if they seem to recover from it. Also phone an ambulance if someone has a seizure which lasts more than three minutes.

- Has a severe allergic reaction. Administer their adrenaline auto-injector (if they have one) and then phone an ambulance immediately.

- Is seriously burnt. For a child or an elderly person with a burn severe enough to need dressing, put the burn under cool running water and call an ambulance. Keep cooling the burn until the paramedics arrive and look out for signs of shock. For a fit adult with a burn, cool it under water for at least 10 minutes – longer if it is still hurting – then apply a burns dressing or loosely cover with cling film and transfer them for immediate medical attention.

- Has fallen from a height, been hit by something travelling at speed (like a car) or been hit with force whilst doing combat or contact sport and there is a possibility of a spinal injury. If they are conscious, keep them completely still and get an ambulance on the way. If they are on their back, unconscious and breathing and you are concerned about their airway, very carefully roll them into the recovery position and phone an ambulance. If they are unconscious and not breathing, start CPR.

Take someone to A&E if they have:

- A fever and are floppy and lethargic

- Severe abdominal pain

- A cut that is gaping or losing a lot of blood, an amputated finger or if they have something embedded in a wound

- A leg or arm injury and can't use the limb

- Swallowed poison or tablets and are not showing any adverse effects (111 can give you advice from the poisons database). If someone has swallowed something poisonous and is behaving strangely/experiencing other symptoms, call an ambulance immediately.

Go to your family doctor for other less serious and non-life-threatening medical concerns. Contact your GP or phone 111 for medical advice.

How to phone an ambulance

Phoning an ambulance is something people assume is second nature. However, in a highly stressful situation, it is easy to find your mind has gone blank. Emergency telephone numbers are different worldwide; you'll get through to the emergency services operator in the UK with 999 and with 112 throughout Europe. The number is 911 in the USA and 000 in Australia. They will ask you which service you require – police, fire or ambulance.

The operator will need to know exactly where you are, so use reference points, landmarks, ask locals or use google maps and give as much information as you can to help them to establish your exact location.

Use speaker phone so you can continue to provide first aid treatment whilst talking to the emergency services. Do what they advise.

They will need to know:
- Your name
- The telephone number you are calling from
- Your location (including postcode if possible)
- The type of accident
- The number of casualties
- The approximate ages of casualties
- Whether the casualties are conscious, unconscious and breathing, or not breathing
- Any other relevant information (such as whether they are taking medication)

If it is a life-threatening emergency, tell the emergency services immediately.

The emergency services will want to work through their algorithm of questions to classify your call. If your call is serious, they will already have dispatched the ambulance, but still need to collate all the information to feed through to the medical responders.

The effect of ageing on our brain, body and how we might react in a medical emergency:

It is of critical importance everyone does their utmost to prevent accidents occurring in the first place and quickly spot and treat any deterioration in health that could result in a hospital admission. When older people become incapacitated following an accident and are admitted to hospital or put on bed rest for any length of time, they can quickly deteriorate and become institutionalised and immobile. An elderly patient will lose 10% of their body mass every week they lie in bed. It is therefore vital they are always encouraged to mobilise as soon as possible. How many times have we heard stories of someone living a fulfilled and active life at home until that fall?!

Falls from less than 2 metres, which would not generally cause serious injury for younger people, represent a leading cause of major trauma for people over the age of 70.

Elderly people are more prone to serious injury from slighter impact as they become less resilient, have reduced physiological reserve*, may suffer from pre-existing medical conditions** and might be affected by unwanted side effects of prescribed medication. In addition, an older skeleton is more brittle and vulnerable to trauma and it is far more likely that an older person will incur broken bones when they fall.

*Physiological reserve is the excess capacity in organs and biological systems that gives us stamina when we are younger. That enables us to push limits when we need to, to run for a bus, climb a mountain or even hold on when we are bursting for a pee! This additional capacity, flexibility and adaptability steadily declines as we get older. As cells deteriorate or die with advancing age, the excess is lost at different rates from different systems. Because we are talking about excess capacity that we normally don't need or use, the loss of this physiological reserve can suddenly become apparent when someone older is involved in an accident and is unable to cope.

**Pre-existing medical conditions:
For example, declining nerve function in diabetics makes people more prone to soft tissue injuries and amputations as the lack of sensation means they may not appreciate the extent of an injury.

Hypoglycaemia and hypothermia affect clotting, meaning people with low blood sugar, or those with a low body temperature are more likely to bleed and are harder to stabilise.

Medication:

Aspirin and warfarin affect non-vitamin k coagulation and make people more prone to bleeding.

Beta blockers, commonly prescribed to reduce blood pressure mean that an elderly person may not exhibit classic signs of shock and early warning signs may be missed.

When someone is experiencing severe shock, the body's autonomic nervous system should take over and cause the blood vessels at the extremities to shut down and divert blood to the vital organs. The heart should beat faster, and blood pressure drop. In an older person, this response may not occur as swiftly; as the autonomic system is slower, the blood vessels may not constrict as quickly, and the ventricles of their heart may be thickened and less able to cope with the increased demand. This may consequently mask the early classic symptoms of shock meaning health professionals may miss opportunities to treat them promptly.

Changes to the older respiratory system:

As people age, the chest wall loses its flexibility and becomes increasingly rigid. Therefore, older people do not have the respiratory reserves of a younger person, a loss of muscle mass in the lungs, reduced alveolar gas exchange because the blood vessels are less efficient and a reduced central nervous system response to any build-up of carbon dioxide in the blood, means an elderly person may not show an increased respiratory rate when they are in distress. Consequently, first aiders and health professionals may miss early warning signs that the person is in respiratory distress or in shock.

From the age of 30 the brain begins to shrink and increases in vascular fragility. Minor infections, injuries and pain can consequently lead to acute confusion and disorientation in older people. If someone suddenly becomes confused it is extremely common for it to be due to a urinary tract, or some other infection. However, acute confusion or any deterioration should always be swiftly investigated as it could be caused by a stroke or some other neurological problem.

It has been suggested that due to the increasing vulnerability of an older brain, it would be sensible to call the emergency services for all head injuries in over 65s.

In older people the skin also thins and becomes more friable (delicate and prone to injury). They are more prone to cuts and minor abrasions, and these injuries are often difficult to heal and may ulcerate. Because the sensation may be dulled, older people are often unaware they have hurt themselves, their skin is often so thin (particularly on their shins) that it becomes papery and the slightest knock can cause it to bleed.

The same reduced sensation and thinning of the skin means older people are more susceptible to burns. Being too close to a radiator or using a hot water bottle can lead to an older person experiencing severe burns.

The success rate for treating older people admitted to hospital is really encouraging: with 32% of over 65s admitted to hospital making a good recovery.

Understanding and managing medication:

As people get older they may need to take more medication. Older people are more prone to aches and pains - for which they usually take tablets - and many develop illnesses that require prescription medication to control and manage symptoms.

Older bodies take longer to respond to, absorb and metabolise medicines and the medicines themselves may react with one another which can increase side effects, or affect their potency.

Changes in body weight can influence the amount of medicine needed and how long they remain in the body. The circulation system may slow down, which can affect how fast drugs get to the liver and kidneys. The liver and kidneys may also work more slowly, affecting the way a drug breaks down and is removed from the body. This means medicines may stay in the body longer and cause more severe side effects if doses are not properly adjusted and monitored. Because of these and other changes in the body as we age, there is also a higher risk of drug interactions in older adults.

Physicians should be cautious when prescribing for the elderly and initially start prescribing a lower dose, monitor closely and gradually increase as needed. Because of the slowing in the metabolising of medication older people may require different intervals and durations of treatment. The longer an individual is on a drug, the greater the likelihood of an adverse reaction. The effects of a harmful drug reaction can appear as an isolated symptom such as drowsiness or as a group of symptoms such as depression and confusion.

1. **Older people take more medicines**—prescription, over-the-counter (OTC) and supplements—than any other age group.

2. **Older adults often use multiple medicines**, increasing the risk of drug interactions, mix-ups and the potential for harmful side effects.

3. **The liver and kidneys my cease to be as effective at metabolising the medication.** This decreased function can affect the way a medicine works, is absorbed, broken down and removed from the body. Therefore, medicines may stay in the body longer and cause more severe side effects if doses are not properly adjusted.

4. **Age-related changes to the body** such as weight loss or gain, alteration in body fluid and increased fatty tissue can alter the way drugs are distributed and concentrated in the body.

5. **Increased sensitivity to many medicines is more common** in older adults.

6. **Impaired memory and hearing and vision loss can make it more difficult** to understand and remember medicine instructions, especially for those who are taking multiple medications. Declining eyesight, grip strength, mobility and memory lapses all affect the ability to safely take medication as prescribed.

7. **Older adults are often under the care of different specialists:** this can make it more difficult to track medicines and identify drug interactions, harmful doses, and unnecessary or ineffective medicines.

Tips to avoid medication problems

Be actively involved in understanding health conditions and prescribed medications. Talk with the healthcare providers, ask questions, read trustworthy and reputable online sites, join health support groups. It is important that everyone involved in the care of the individual is active in understanding their condition, medication and all the options available to treat them.

Have medication and/or a list of medications available at all times to show health professionals in case an accident occurs.

Write a medication list that includes:

- Names of all medications, including any Over the Counter (OTC) medications, dietary supplements and herbal remedies

- The doctor who prescribed each prescription medication

- The purpose of each medication or the symptoms the medication is supposed to treat

- How often and at what dose (amount) to take

- Should they be taken on a full or empty stomach?

- When repeat prescriptions are required

Be sure to update the list if taking something new, a medicine is stopped, or the dose is changed. GPs and pharmacists should review all medications regularly. Remind them of any allergies or problems encountered with certain medicines. Don't stop taking prescribed medicine without checking with them first.

It is also important to know the following about each drug taken:

- Medication name, exact spelling, purpose, and whether it is the brand name or a generic substitution (many medications have similar sounding names).

- The medication's side effects or drug interactions, and what to do if they occur. Report any new symptoms to your physician.

- How and when to take the medication (i.e. on an empty stomach, after meals or at bed time etc.).

- How long the medication is to be continued and if any blood tests are required for periodic monitoring.

- What to do if you miss or forget a dosage.

- How to store your medications - in a refrigerator or at room temperature...

Read the Patient Medicine Information leaflets (provided in the packaging of the prescription medicine.) These provide important information to help understand the medication and avoid problems. Such as:

- What the medicine has been prescribed for

- How to take the medicine correctly (how often you should take it and at what amount or dose and whether it should be on a full or empty stomach)

- Possible side effects to watch out for and any interaction with other medications or food substances – whether it could cause drowsiness etc.

- Interactions with alcohol

- Warnings. This includes who shouldn't take the medicine, serious side effects that mean medication should be stopped and an appointment made urgently with the doctor and information as to who is at increased risks of side effects.

- Storage instructions

Dietary and drug interactions

Be aware of possible dietary interactions. For example, grapefruit juice can increase the absorption of cholesterol-lowering statins. It can also affect the way the body metabolises various drugs, resulting in a higher or lower blood concentration. Many medications are affected in this way, including antihistamines, blood pressure drugs, thyroid replacement drugs, birth control and stomach acid-blocking drugs. It's best to avoid or significantly restrict consumption of grapefruit juice when taking these medications. Grapefruit also interacts with calcium channel blockers prescribed for lowering blood pressure and can totally nullify their effects. It is also thought to interact with drugs for erectile dysfunction, increasing their potency and making men more prone to serious side effects.

Caffeine can cause problems with some bronchodilators and asthma medication.

Warfarin (Coumadin) is a blood-thinning medication that helps treat and prevent blood clots. Eating foods rich in vitamin K can make warfarin less effective. The highest concentrations of vitamin K are found in green leafy vegetables such as kale, spinach, Brussels sprouts and broccoli. It is not necessary to avoid leafy vegetables, but important to keep your intake consistent as your dose will have been calculated based on the diet you were on when the warfarin was prescribed.

ACE inhibitors, commonly prescribed to lower blood pressure, can increase the amount of potassium in the body. Too much potassium can be harmful, causing an irregular heartbeat and heart palpitations. Avoid eating large amounts of foods high in potassium, such as bananas, oranges, green leafy vegetables, and salt substitutes that contain potassium.

Digoxin absorption can be affected by dietary fibre and so should be taken an hour before or 2 hours after a meal. Herbs can also affect digoxin; ginseng can elevate blood levels of digoxin by as much as 75%, while St. John's Wort can decrease them by 25%.

Anti-thyroid drugs work by preventing iodine absorption in the stomach. A diet high in iodine requires higher doses of anti-thyroid drugs, increasing the chance of problematic side effects such as rashes, hives, and liver disease. The richest dietary sources of iodine are seafood and seaweed, such as kelp and nori and green vegetables such as cabbage. Thyroxine can be affected by soya bean and walnuts.

Use one pharmacy to build a helpful relationship with the pharmacist and keep prescription records in one place. This enables the pharmacist to regularly monitor medications and inform you about potential drug interactions. Many pharmacists can renew prescriptions automatically and can arrange for someone else to collect medication.

Store medicines safely. Check expiration dates. Keep all medication in its original packaging - bottle, box or tube - so the dosage and directions are always close at hand. Keep medicines out of the sight and reach of pets and children. Ensure you move them off bedside or breakfast tables when grandchildren come to visit. Be mindful of medication within your handbag when visiting little ones and never share prescription medicines or take others' medications.

Take a friend or family member with you when visiting the doctor or a hospital specialist. Write down all the issues to discuss before the appointment and include a list of all the medication that is currently being taken and any previously prescribed which you have discontinued due to side effects etc...

Alcohol may interact with many medications

Drinking alcohol when taking a prescription can present a significant health risk. As we get older our liver may struggle to cope with alcohol and medication. Many prescription medications can interact with alcohol and cause potentially dangerous adverse effects. Some prescription medications may not work as intended when combined with alcohol, some may not work at all, and some may become harmful. Consult a health care professional for additional guidance.

Driving and prescription medication

Be careful when driving and operating machinery when taking prescription medication as it may cause dizziness, drowsiness or altered vision. If affected, cease driving immediately and consult a health professional.

Diabetic medication can be difficult to manage accurately

Sometimes medication can cause low blood sugar, which may lead to confusion or falls, and it has been linked to a fast decline brain function. Particular care needs to be taken with older diabetics; drugs that lower blood sugar have caused many medication-related hospitalisations.

Caution with Beta Blockers

Beta blockers can be used alone or with other medicines to treat high blood pressure. They are also used to prevent angina (chest pain) and treat heart attacks. They work by slowing the heart rate and relaxing the blood vessels, so the heart doesn't have to work as hard to pump blood. It is important that people understand they must not stop taking a beta blocker without talking to their doctor. Stopping a beta blocker suddenly can lead to chest pain, an irregular heartbeat or heart attack. Doctors usually recommend decreasing your dose gradually.

Blood pressure medication can often be prescribed at a dose that brings blood pressure much lower than the goal pressure. This can result in light-headedness or even falls when an older person stands up.

Risks in Using Multiple Medications

Prescription medications can improve the symptoms of a disorder and improve quality of life. However, they can also cause potentially dangerous side effects. Always report any unusual or new symptoms to your health care provider.

It is important to consult a health care provider before changing any prescription medication dosage.

Common medications in the elderly and their possible side effects

Medications listed below should be prescribed to older people with additional caution. Those taking these medications should be monitored closely to spot any side effects early and, if necessary, look to change treatments.

Side effects being mentioned does not mean they will occur. Many of these medications are well-tolerated by people of all ages.

Medication – generic name	Possible problems/common side effects
Sleeping tablets such as Benzodiazepines, Barbiturates (used to treat anxiety, panic attacks and problems sleeping), **Examples:** Diazepam, Temazepam, Flurazepam, Chlordiazepoxide, Alprazolam	Confusion, sleepiness, greater incidence of falls
Antidepressants (used to treat depression) **Examples:** Amitriptyline (may be prescribed for Parkinsonian tremor) Doxepin Imipramine	Confusion, drowsiness, hypotension (low blood pressure which can lead to dizziness when getting up), falls, and urinary retention (the inability to empty your bladder making you more at risk of urinary tract infections).
Antipsychotic Agents (used for psychiatric disorders) Chlorpromazine Thioridazine Haloperidol	Confusion, drowsiness, hypotension, increased risk of falls, urinary retention, Parkinsonism (involuntary shaking and twitching). Can also make people more sensitive to sunlight.
Antihistamines (used to treat sinus problems and allergies) Diphenhydramine (Benadryl) Hydroxyzine – also used for anti-anxiety	Confusion, drowsiness, hypotension, increased risk of falls, and urinary retention (inability to empty bladder), sleep disturbances. Hydroxyzine often interacts with other medications and alcohol.
Antiemetics (used to relieve nausea) Promethazine Prochlorperazine Thiethylperazine	Confusion, drowsiness, hypotension, increased risk of falls, urinary retention, Parkinsonism (involuntary tremors and rigidity), involuntary movement (tardive dyskinaesia)

Analgesics (painkillers) Codeine based medication Pethidine	Constipation, confusion, sedation
Antiparkinsonian (used to treat Parkinson's disease) Carbidopa-Levodopa	Confusion, dizziness, hypotension, increase in cardiovascular toxicity which can damage the heart
Cardiovascular drugs (used to treat heart and blood vessels) Digoxin – for cardiac arrhythmias Warfarin – anti-clotting agent	Nausea, vomiting, anorexia, weight loss. Warfarin – bleeding and clotting problems (requires close monitoring through prothrombin test and frequently interacts with antibiotics and other medication)
Antispasmodic drugs (used to prevent or relieve spasms usually in the bowel and bladder and used for Parkinson's) Dicyclomine Hyoscyamine Pro-Banthine	Dry mouth, constipation, urinary retention, delirium, can supress breathing and cause difficulty sleeping
Urinary Incontinence drugs Oxybutynin Tolterodine	Dry mouth, constipation, urinary retention, confusion

Sensible lifestyle changes that can reduce the reliance on medication

Simple changes to the way we live can sometimes mean we can avoid medication. It is sensible to try non-pharmacological approaches and healthy lifestyle changes to manage a condition before resorting to pills. However, never make any changes to medication without discussing it with the doctor first.

Alternatives to taking sleeping tablets:

- Monitor sleep patterns and try and adopt a regular routine. Go to bed and wake up at a fixed time.
- Have a bath or milky drink before bedtime
- Use lavender to help promote a natural sleep
- Avoid caffeine after 1 p.m. and if possible remove it from your diet altogether.
- Increase exercise and avoid daytime napping.
- Avoid alcohol close to bed time.
- Don't use mobile phones or other gadgets emitting blue light before bedtime.

Alternatives to taking laxatives:

- Eat a high fibre diet and plenty of fruit.
- Drink plenty of water.
- Exercise regularly.
- Identify medications causing constipation – codeine based painkillers can often lead to constipation.

Alternatives to taking medication for urinary incontinence:

- There are many proven bladder training and pelvic exercises – GPs can recommend specialists to help.
- Visit the bathroom every two hours while awake.
- Treat urinary infections promptly with antibiotics.
- If night time incontinence is a problem or getting up in the night is an issue, avoid drinking a couple of hours before bed.
- Discuss the problem with the GP as there may be a treatable medical reason for the incontinence.

Tips to help remember what medication to take and when

It is extremely common for older people to make mistakes with their medication. According to the Department of Health, 55% of the elderly are "non-compliant" with their prescription drugs orders, meaning they don't use medication in the way it was prescribed and this often leads to complications and hospital admissions.

- There are many helpful boxes and organisers (with the days of the week written on each compartment) to help organise medication.
- Ask the doctor or pharmacist for help simplifying and streamlining daily medication.
- For drugs taken several times a day, there may be a once-a-day option.
- Ask whether a drug can be stopped, and a non-drug treatment tried instead.
- Pharmacists can often recommend ways to safely adjust when and how medications are taken.

Swallowing Problems

Swallowing can become more difficult as we get older and often particularly the swallowing of tablets. Crushing, chewing and breaking tablets can cause problems as long-acting medicines will be released too quickly and this will affect the way the medication is absorbed and metabolised. Sometimes there are alternatives, such as a liquid or sugar-coated version or different formulation. Consult a doctor and pharmacist if swallowing the medication is a problem.

- Never crush, chew, break or mix the tablet or capsule in fluid unless the doctor or pharmacist says it is okay to do so.
- Ask for liquids. If someone has trouble swallowing medicines, ask the doctor or pharmacist if there is a liquid alternative.

Tips to prevent common accidents and falls

Falls are the most common cause of injury-related deaths in people over the age of 75. Over 4,500 people in England and Wales died as a result of a fall in 2015. Every year, following a fall, nearly a third of a million people need hospital treatment. Many older people who suffer from falls never fully recover from either the physical or psychological impact of their injuries.

Although the fall itself may not cause a serious injury, if the casualty is unable to get up following their fall, they are more likely to suffer hypothermia or pressure sores. Most accidents in the elderly result from falls from stairs or steps.

As we get older we are more prone to lose our balance through sudden movements, e.g. getting out of bed or a chair too quickly. This is often more apparent if taking medication for high blood pressure. Getting up very slowly and bringing the head up last can reduce the dizzying effects of postural hypotension. Eyesight is also unlikely to be as good as it was, particularly in low light and so it is even more important to avoid tripping hazards.

Eat well: People should try and eat a balanced diet that includes calcium-rich food, such as cheese and milk to strengthen bones, and oily fish, like sardines and tuna, which contain vitamin D. Low levels of vitamin D can increase risk of falls. Taking supplements may be helpful. GPs and pharmacists can advise.

Exercise: There is increasing evidence on the importance of regular exercise in reducing the likelihood of falls. Exercises that strengthen the core muscles and help improve balance have been shown to be extremely helpful. GPs also have the opportunity to refer at risk patients to specific exercise programmes designed to help balance, improve stamina and general fitness and work on core body strength and posture. These classes have an excellent success rate in reducing falls and are also good fun and an opportunity to meet new people.

Medical conditions can also make falls more likely:

- Arthritis and similar conditions can weaken and stiffen muscles.
- Heart conditions or changes in blood pressure can cause people to feel dizzy when getting up too quickly.

- Parkinson's disease can cause tremors and make people less stable.

- Hearing problems can affect balance.

- Side effects of some medications cause dizziness or drowsiness and make you less aware of your surroundings.

- We are less able to metabolise alcohol as we get older, thus it can have a greater potency.

- Urgency for the loo can also make it more likely for someone to fall and slip following an episode of incontinence. If this is an issue, there are things GPs can do to help.

The NHS have a helpful falls risk assessment tool to help assess how at risk someone is of falling.

Advice to prevent falls

- As you get older, your body may not respond as quickly as it used to. Older people may need to take a little more time to get up, to allow their body to adjust to the movement and prevent dizziness and stumbling.

- Items should not be left on the stairs, it is so easy to trip over them.

- Replace damaged carpet and avoid repetitive carpet patterns that can affect perception and make it more difficult to see individual stairs.

- Ensure landings, stairs and hallways are well lit with two-way light switches

- Ensure banisters are secure and sturdy. Two easy-grip handrails gives more stability.

- Floors and surfaces should be as clear as possible. Worn rugs, slippery floors and paths, uneven surfaces, trailing flexes, and items left lying around make falling far more likely.

- Pay attention to footwear. Ill-fitting shoes, older shoes that have lost their grip and stretched slippers often contribute to a fall.

- Grab rails and places to sit down in the bathroom and kitchen can be helpful when feeling dizzy.

- Floors should be cleaned carefully to ensure they're not slippery. Any spillages should be immediately and thoroughly removed.

- Sometimes urgency to get to the toilet can cause people to fall and incontinence can cause people to slip. If urgency or incontinence is a problem, the doctor may be able to refer to a special clinic for help.

Having a fall could be an indicator of a treatable underlying health problem. It is sensible to make an appointment with the GP for a check-up and possibly ask for a referral to an NHS Falls Clinic where they can further investigate and help instigate measures to prevent further falls. There's physiotherapy, specific muscle-strengthening exercise classes and lots of advice and support available.

It is sensible to have a charged mobile phone accessible at all times and consider installing a community alarm system to be able to quickly summon help if needed.

There is helpful technology available such as Telecare technology which sends an alert to a relative, carer or call centre if someone gets up from a bed or chair and fails to return in a set time.

Other common injuries in the older population

Burns

As we get older skin becomes thinner, delicate and more sensitive to heat. In addition, if someone has peripheral nerve damage, it may mean they do not feel pain and are not immediately aware that they have burnt themselves. Reflexes are not as quick in older age. Older people may also feel the cold more and are tempted to go to extremes to keep warm.

Measures to prevent burns:

Fit oven shelf guards; easily available from many online and mail order companies, these protect you from burns when removing things from the oven.

Get a kettle with a short or curly flex and ensure it is not somewhere it can be knocked or accidentally pulled over.

Consider buying a smaller kettle and only boil as much water as you need

Hot drinks should ideally be cooled before transporting and consuming them. Trolleys are often a safer option for people to transport hot cups of tea and tea pots around the house.

Take care when microwaving; ensure food and drink is properly stirred to avoid scalds from hot spots.

Hot water bottles should never be filled with boiling water and should always be covered. Beds should not be positioned close to radiators. Care should be taken with heated under-blankets and all wiring and heating appliances should be regularly checked to ensure there isn't a fire risk.

The fire service can be contacted to come and help with a fire risk assessment, to check smoke alarms and generally ensure there are no obvious fire hazards and there is easy exit in case of fire.

Tips to prevent choking:

Choking often occurs when someone talks, sniffs or laughs whilst eating a meal.

Older people begin to develop difficulties swallowing and this can make them more prone to choking. If they have dental problems, they may experience pain when chewing and this can mean they try and swallow food before it has been properly broken down, making them more likely to choke. To avoid this, encourage them to cut their food up and chew thoroughly.

If choking is a repeated problem, talk to the family doctor as there are specialists who can assess the situation and help.

Bleeding and skin ulceration:

Older people's skin is thinner and can become papery, particularly on the shins and arms. It is very easy for them to catch themselves on things and it can take a long time to heal. If an elderly person is on warfarin, they are also more likely to bleed, and when someone is extremely cold, blood takes longer to clot.

Look for hazards at shin-level and ensure they are made safe. Older people may need help keeping their finger and toe nails short; long nails can lead to them injuring themselves.

Be vigilant for early signs of pressure sores. If people are sitting or lying for prolonged lengths of time without moving themselves sufficiently they will develop pressure sores. Incontinence will also make this more likely. It is important to discuss this with the GP and they can help with referrals for pressure-relieving mattresses, cushions and other devices to prevent pressure sores occurring in the first place.

Be very careful to avoid injuries from shopping trolleys, pushchairs and wheelchairs. They can easily rupture varicose veins if they hit an elderly person in the calf.

If someone does hurt themselves and it is taking a long time to heal, they should see their GP to ensure the injury is assessed properly and to avoid long-term leg ulcers.

Part 2

Action in an emergency

Managing an incident
Assess the situation and make safe

Give emergency aid

Get help

Deal with the aftermath

You should always start by checking for DANGER – you don't know what has injured them and if you are injured as well, you won't be able to help them.

You need to keep yourself safe the whole time, ensure that in addition to a check at the beginning, you make sure you don't put yourself at risk at any point. Keep as calm as possible and keep things simple. Always treat what you can see.

Priorities of Treatment

- Preserve life

- Prevent the condition worsening

- Promote recovery

When you are dealing with a serious incident, it is crucially important that you prioritise any life-threatening conditions and treat those first.

35

1 Breathing

This is your number one priority, if they are not breathing and you don't do anything about it, they will die!

2 Bleeding and Burns

Both can be life-threatening conditions. Providing the casualty is breathing, your next priority is to stop bleeding and treat burns, before being distracted by anything else.

3 Broken Bones

These are rarely life-threatening and can prove a distraction from more serious priorities.

Preparing for an emergency

Things to think about before something happens:

It is very helpful to think in advance about how you would manage a medical emergency.

1. Make sure you have a fully-charged mobile phone with you and have close neighbours' numbers on there as well as your next of kin. Swap keys with neighbours and have their details in case you have an accident in the home and need their help.

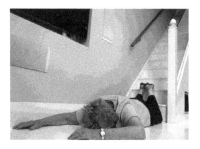

2. Find out where the nearest hospital is and what specialties they have. Learn where your closest out of hours chemist is and have their telephone number and opening hours to hand.

3. Just a few minutes on Google can supply you with these numbers and they should be written up and placed prominently by the phone, so the information is to hand. It is useful to have them laminated as a credit card-sized document to keep with you as well, should something happen when you're out and about.

Helpful information

- Carers should ensure they have detailed medical information including prescribed medication for conditions such as asthma, diabetes, anaphylaxis, sickle cell, heart conditions and any other relevant medical conditions. This information should be stored securely but easily accessible in case of an emergency. They should also have contact numbers for guardians and next of kin.

- Medication such as asthma pumps and adrenaline auto-injectors should be clearly marked and remain safe but accessible for urgent use.

- If a casualty is injured outdoors, it is important to try and insulate them from the ground if possible and cover them to keep them warm.

- Ensure that there is an appropriately stocked first aid kit to hand.

Role of the First Aider

1. As a first aider it is important to keep as calm as possible and use your first aid training. Staying calm evades panic and has been proven to be hugely important. It can make a massive difference, particularly if a casualty is showing signs of shock, choking or having an asthma attack.

2. Assess the situation quickly and call for help immediately if necessary.

3. Keep yourself and others safe and protected; remove any dangers and minimise the risk of infection.

4. Prioritise casualties and injuries, treating the most serious first.

The Primary Survey – How to help in an Emergency

A primary survey is a fast and systematic way to find and treat any life-threatening conditions in order of priority.

Danger

- Check for electrical cables, broken glass, chemicals and ensure you do not put yourself at risk.

- If the casualty is a stranger, approach with caution.

- If there is any danger remove it. If the casualty is being electrocuted, the electricity should be turned off at the mains before they are touched, otherwise you could be electrocuted as well.

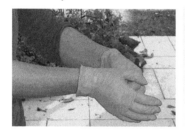 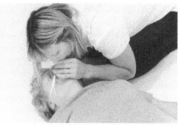

Wear gloves if possible   Use a face shield to resuscitate

Make sure everyone is safe. You are of no help to anyone if you become an additional casualty.

Only on the rare occasions that the danger cannot be removed should you move the casualty instead. Examples of this are fire, flood, danger of explosion, chemical spills etc.

Response

To establish whether a casualty is conscious:

1. Shout assertively and ask them to open their eyes.

2. Tap/shake them gently or give them a short painful stimulus, such as a pinch on their ear or nail bed.

3. If there is no response when you pinch one ear, pinch the other, in case they have a weakness down one side.

4. If you get any response at all, you know they are breathing and therefore their heart is beating.

5. If there is hardly any response and they are drifting in and out of consciousness, if you have to leave them, put them in the recovery position first.

6. If there is **no** response, **shout for help**. Do not leave the casualty at this stage. If there are multiple casualties, the quiet ones take priority as they may be unconscious and need urgent treatment.

How to assess someone's level of consciousness

Alert – Fully responsive and conscious

Voice – Responds to you when you speak or shout to them

Pain – Groans or responds in some way when you pinch them

Unresponsive – Not conscious enough to keep their own airway clear.

Someone is considered to be unresponsive if they do not react at all when you speak to them or hurt them.

Most common causes of unconsciousness (unresponsiveness)

FISH SHAPED

Fainting
Inability to maintain body temperature/imbalance of heat (e.g. heat stroke, hypothermia)
Shock
Head injury

Stroke
Heart attack
Asphyxia – lack of oxygen caused by an airway blockage (e.g. suffocation, drowning, asthma, choking, strangulation, gas poisoning)
Poisoning
Epilepsy/fitting
Diabetes

Airway

When you are unconscious/unresponsive most of your muscles relax and go floppy. Your tongue is a huge muscle attached to your bottom jaw. If you are unconscious and lying on your back, the back of your tongue will flop back and block your airway, making you unable to breathe. In addition, your oesophagus (the tube from your throat to your stomach) and the sphincter (valve at the top of your stomach) relax and remain open. This means the contents of your stomach may trickle up and drip into your lungs. This is called passive vomiting.

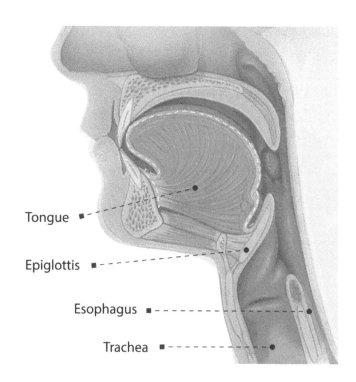

Tongue

Epiglottis

Esophagus

Trachea

| *Throat Anatomy*

Note: If someone is unconscious and you are aware of the presence of vomit (because you can see it, smell it or they are gurgling), immediately roll them onto their side to empty them. If there is vomit at the back of their throat, they will be unable to breathe in.

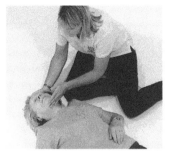

To open someone's airway (lifting the tongue from the back of the throat)

Tilt the head and lift the chin. Try this yourself; you will find that if your head is all the way back and you push your chin forward, you are unable to swallow.

Never try and pull someone's tongue or put your fingers down to clear an airway.

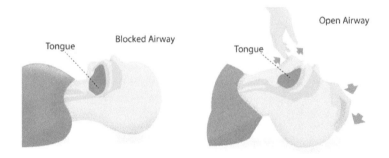

Tilting their head and lifting their chin forward will automatically move their tongue away from the back of their throat so their airway is clear.

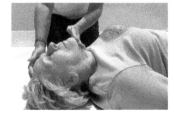

If the person is unresponsive and breathing, the only way to keep their airway open and clear is to put them on their side (in the recovery position). This will mean their tongue flops forward and any vomit is able to drain from their mouth.

41

Breathing

Just after their heart 'stops', a casualty may appear to be breathing when they are not. These breaths are called "agonal gasps" and are a reflex action from the lungs, **not** effective breathing. If there are less than 2 breaths in a 10 second period, the person is not breathing sufficiently, and you will need to start CPR.

If in doubt, always start CPR; it is better to try and resuscitate someone unnecessarily than not to resuscitate someone that has stopped breathing.

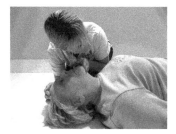 Tilt their head and lift their chin to open the airway. Then place the side of your face above their mouth and nose and look down the body to check for breathing. Look for movement of the chest, listen for the sound of breathing and feel their breath on your cheek for up to 10 seconds and you should see at least 2 breaths.

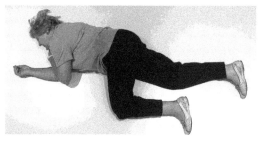

| *Recovery position*

1. If they are unresponsive and breathing normally, put them in the recovery position immediately.

2. If someone is unresponsive and not breathing normally, start CPR.

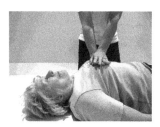 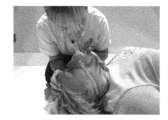

Action in an emergency

Unresponsive and Breathing

If someone is unconscious but you're sure they are breathing, the best way to keep the airway open is to roll them onto their side, in the recovery position. This will make their tongue flop forward and allow the contents of their stomach to drain.

Recovery position

Ideally, the casualty should not be on their front as this puts the weight of their body on their lungs and it is not as easy to breathe. To avoid this, bend their knee to 90 degrees in order to support them on their side. Once they are in the recovery position, keep checking they are breathing by holding the back of your hand in front of their mouth.

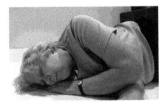

It is important that the head is angled over sufficiently to allow any vomit to drain. Providing there is no possibility of a spinal injury, once on their side, tilt the head back slightly to further open the airway.

How to put someone in the recovery position

If someone is unconscious but breathing, and lying on their back, their tongue will flop to the back of their throat, the contents of their stomach will drain upwards and they will not be able to breathe. To stop this happening, they need to be rolled into the recovery position as quickly as possible.

The following method shows you how to put someone into the recovery position if you are on your own – even if you think they could have a spinal injury.

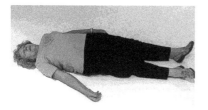 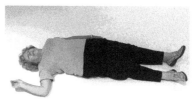

If you are not worried about a spinal injury, or if they are very heavy, you can just use the knee as a lever to pull them over - there is no need to support their head and neck. If you are worried about the possibility of a spinal injury and you have other people to help, it is best to log roll them to keep the spine in line.

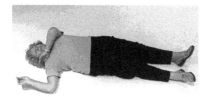 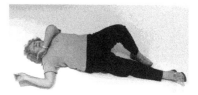

1. Move the arm closest to you out of the way. Use your hand which is closest to their head to hold their other hand and put this onto the side of their cheek to support the head and neck as you turn them.

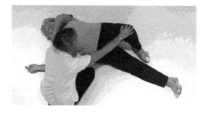

2. Use your other hand to lift up the outside of their knee. Then use this as a lever to pull them over.

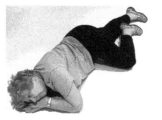

3. Pull the knee to the floor, whilst supporting their head and neck with your other hand.

Pull their bent knee upwards into a running position to stabilise their body. Ensure they are over enough to make their tongue flop forward and allow the contents of their stomach to drain out.

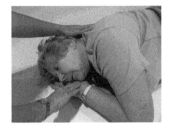

If you are not worried about a possible spinal injury, tilt their head back slightly to ensure the airway is properly open. If you are worried about a possible neck injury, just ensure they are rolled over enough for any vomit to drain.

Keep checking that they are breathing.

Get the emergency services on the way if they haven't been called before.

Secondary Survey

- First complete the primary survey; prioritising and treating any life-threatening injuries. Then you can begin the secondary survey; a top-to-toe, detailed examination of what is wrong.

- If someone is unconscious, the secondary survey should be carried out with them in the recovery position and they should be moved as little as possible. If there is any obvious core body or head injury, they should be placed on their injured side.

- Once they are in the recovery position and their airway is open, check for any other injuries. First look for watery blood coming from either ear and feel their chest to see if both lungs are moving equally. Look for any other serious injuries, such as bleeding or burns.

- Keep checking that they are still breathing – that is always your top priority. If the casualty is conscious, talk to them calmly and reassure them.

Ask open questions to find out what is wrong. Examples of useful questions:

- **What happened?** This allows you to find out more about how the accident happened; helping you make a proper assessment of the situation. It can also help establish whether they have hit their head and are suffering from any short-term memory loss.

- **Where does it hurt most?** This helps to work out exactly where they are injured.

- **Can you take a deep breath?** This helps to work out how seriously they are injured and whether their breathing is involved.

Heart Attacks

Fatty deposits and plaques cause atheroma that builds up in coronary arteries and reduces the lumen of the artery, meaning that blood flows slower through the vessel.

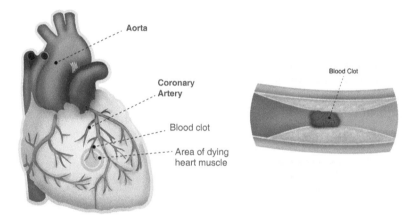

A heart attack is often caused by a clot forming in this slow-moving blood and this then blocks that coronary artery completely, depriving the heart muscle of oxygen; causing that part of the heart to stop working properly.

The severity of the heart attack and symptoms experienced depends on how large an artery is affected, where in the heart the blockage has occurred and how much of the heart muscle is affected.

If the signs of a heart attack are recognised quickly enough and the casualty is transferred to a specialist Cardiac Unit immediately, they can undergo immediate angioplasty (surgically and mechanically unblocking the blocked artery). This can save the damaged heart muscle by restoring the blood supply.

With a heart attack, you will see the signs and symptoms of someone in shock (i.e. pale, cold, clammy, breathless, blueness, extreme anxiety).

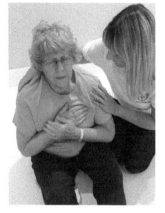

Do not elevate the casualty's legs (as you would normally with someone in shock) as this would put too much strain on the struggling heart and make it harder for them to breathe if they are breathless.

Sit them on the ground in the lazy-W position, with a pillow or something under their legs and help them to sit upright to help their breathing. If this is too difficult for them, just help them to sit down.

Call the emergency services.

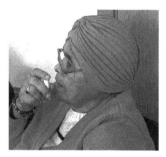

If they have cardiac medication such as a GTN spray, help them to use it.

If this does not work and they have been prescribed a **300mg aspirin,** advise them to **chew it** as it will get into their blood stream more quickly this way.

If they collapse and are unconscious and not breathing, start CPR immediately.

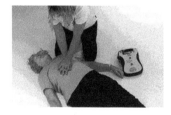

If you have a defibrillator available, open it up and it will start giving you instructions. Dry the casualty's chest and place the pads onto it. Follow the diagrams on the pads to know where to put them.

Ideally one person should be doing CPR while someone else puts the pads on the casualty's chest and concentrates on defibrillating. Do not stop doing CPR until a paramedic arrives and can take over, or the casualty begins to regain consciousness.

47

Angina

Angina is caused by a narrowing of the blood vessels that supply the heart with oxygenated blood. The narrowing is due to a build-up of fatty plaques and deposits on the lining of the artery, which slows down the blood flow.

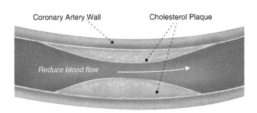

If someone is stressed or exercising, their heart rate speeds up. This means the heart needs more blood and the coronary arteries need to supply the heart with that additional blood. If the coronary arteries are narrowed due to deposits they may not be able to supply enough blood and the heart muscle can develop cramping pain. This results in an Angina attack.

GTN spray is prescribed for Angina. It is sprayed under the tongue and passes through the blood supply to the coronary arteries, dilating blood vessels and allowing blood to pass through more quickly, which relieves the cramping pain.

If someone has not been prescribed GTN, but is having an angina attack, they should begin to feel better if they are able to rest. They should still seek medical attention quickly - even if it does resolve - as having an attack indicates the coronary arteries are quite severely narrowed, and they are at a risk of having a heart attack.

If the pain does not go in less than 10 minutes, they may be having a heart attack.

Unconscious and not breathing

CPR – Cardio Pulmonary Resuscitation

Resuscitation – what exactly are you doing?

1. When you are resuscitating someone, you are acting as a life support machine. When you push on their chest, you are being their heart and when you breathe into them, you are being their lungs. You are keeping their heart and brain full of oxygenated blood, keeping them alive so when the paramedics arrive with a defibrillator they have a good chance of bringing them back to life.

2. **If you are unsure whether or not they are breathing, you will need to start CPR (Cardio Pulmonary Resuscitation).**

Phone for an ambulance.

It is vital to resuscitate if you are unsure. It is much better to attempt to resuscitate someone who doesn't need it, than not to resuscitate someone who does!

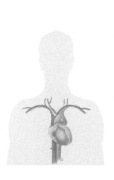 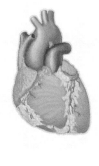

| *Heart Position*

How to perform CPR

1. **When someone collapses and is unresponsive and not breathing, they have residual oxygenated blood remaining in their system. Their heart is no longer working effectively, and it is therefore important to circulate that oxygenated blood by pushing hard and fast on their chest.**

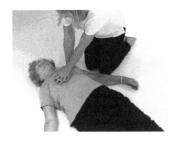

Push on the centre of their chest

Push down 5-6 cm – roughly a third of the depth of their chest

Push at a rate of 115-120 beats per minute – roughly 2 per second

Do 30 compressions then…

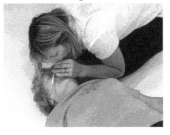

Tilt the head and lift the chin to take the tongue off the back of the airway and hold their nose

Give **2 breaths** – sealing your mouth around theirs and blowing into them like a balloon

2. Make sure their chest rises each time – if it doesn't, try tilting the head a bit more

    If it still won't rise, go straight back to compressions.

3. **Research has shown it takes around 10 compressions to reach sufficient pressure to get the blood circulating to the heart and brain. This is why it is advised you do 30 compressions and then 2 short breaths, to top up their oxygen.**

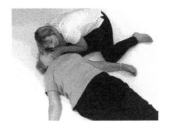 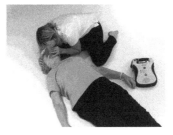

4. **If there is one available, use a face shield to protect yourself.**

5. **Keep going** – you are being a life support machine, keeping them alive!

Do not expect them to regain consciousness and (unless you see very obvious signs of life) keep going until the paramedics are there to help.

If you have someone to share with, do cycles of compressions and breaths and swap every 2 minutes.

If you are on your own, call an ambulance as soon as you realise they are unresponsive and not breathing.

If there is an AED machine around, use it!

Defibrillators (AEDs)

If there is an AED (Automated External Defibrillator) around, use it! A defibrillator is used to give a shock to stop the heart if it is in a shockable rhythm. The heart's own back up system should then re-start the heart back into the desired sinus rhythm. You cannot do any harm, as the machine will not let you deliver a shock to them if they don't need it. The chance of surviving a cardiac arrest jumps from 6% to 74% if a casualty is in a shockable rhythm and receives a shock from a defibrillator within 3 minutes. For every minute's delay there is a further 10% reduction in survival rate. It is vital to act quickly. Defibrillators can be found in many public places in the community and they are extremely easy to use. Open it up and follow the voice prompts.

Hygiene during CPR

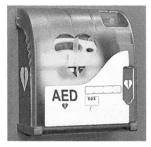 When someone is unconscious, muscles relax and the sphincter muscle above the stomach that retains the contents within the stomach relaxes and opens. It is therefore likely that anything within the casualty's stomach will drain upwards, causing the casualty to passively vomit. This is unpleasant if you are doing mouth-to-mouth resuscitation. You are unlikely to catch anything serious from someone you are resuscitating however, if at all possible, you should use a face shield to protect yourself.

If you do not have a professional mask or face shield, use an improvised face shield – a shirt, scarf or plastic bag with a hole in it. This allows you to resuscitate without it being too intimate and unpleasant, but will not protect you from blood, vomit or infection. If you are unwilling or unable to give mouth-to-mouth, just give chest compressions.

If someone starts gurgling during resuscitation, turn them onto their side immediately, help remove the vomit, give them a wipe, then roll them back to start again.

Compression-only resuscitation

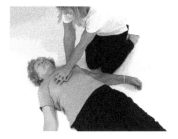

To give someone the best chance, you need to be giving them breaths as well as compressions. Compressions are used to get sufficient pressure in the system to pump the blood to the vital organs; however, that blood needs to be oxygenated to be of any use to the organs. Without breaths, the body will run out of oxygen quickly.

If you are unable or unwilling to give rescue breaths, doing compressions alone will give them 3 or 4 minutes that they would not have otherwise and is much better than not doing anything at all.

Part 3

Choking

Choking occurs when something gets stuck in the back of the throat and blocks the airway. When it is partially blocked the casualty can usually cough and still make noises. When it is totally blocked, the casualty is unable to make any sound at all.

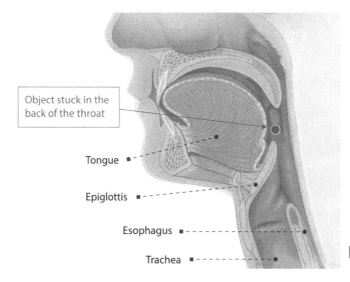

Object stuck in the back of the throat

Tongue

Epiglottis

Esophagus

Trachea

|*Throat Anatomy*

53

How to help if someone is choking

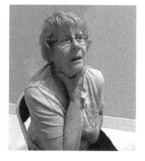

Firstly, check if they are able to cough. Encourage them to do so as people can often clear blockages themselves.

If they are unable to cough:

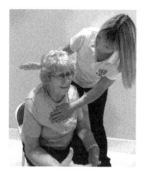

Bend them forward, supporting their chest with one hand and using the flat of your other hand to give a **firm back blow** between the shoulder blades. Check to see if the blockage has cleared before giving another blow.

If the blockage hasn't cleared after five blows, try abdominal thrusts/Heimlich manoeuvre:

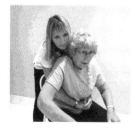

Stand behind them and place one hand in a fist under their rib cage. Use the other hand to pull in and up under their rib cage - in a J-shaped motion - to dislodge the obstruction. Perform abdominal thrusts **up to 5 times,** checking each time to see if the obstruction has cleared. Anyone who has received abdominal thrusts must be seen by a doctor.

If the person is still choking, **call 999** (or 112) and alternate five back blows and five abdominal thrusts until emergency help arrives. **If at any point they become unconscious, start CPR.**

Drowning

Always ensure basic safety around water.

If someone is submerged under the water, but is still conscious, they are not yet drowning. However, if the water is very cold, they may need treatment for mild hypothermia.

Generally, drowning casualties do not **inhale** large amounts of water. Most deaths from drowning are caused from secondary drowning (see below) or from a muscle spasm in the throat that causes the airway to block because of the drowning sensation.

However, drowning casualties do tend to **swallow** large amounts of water and are very likely to vomit as a result. When resuscitating, be aware of this as you may need to turn them onto their side periodically to ensure that they do not inhale and aspirate vomit into their lungs.

Note: lifeguards and those trained in water rescue who have been trained to give rescue breaths before starting compressions, continue with this protocol.

If you are aware that someone is drowning:

1. If they are unconscious in water; remove them as quickly as you can, **but never put yourself in danger.**

2. As soon as you get onto dry land, turn them onto their back and check for breathing. If they are not breathing start resuscitation immediately.

3. Do 30 chest compressions, pushing down hard and fast, followed by 2 rescue breaths.

4. If it is warm and they weren't in the water for very long, they may start to regain consciousness fairly quickly, in which case put them into the recovery position immediately to help them to drain.

5. If it is cold, they are unlikely to come back to life until their body is warm enough.

6. Do 30 compressions to 2 breaths and keep going. Grab a coat or something to put over them.

7. **Call for the emergency services and continue CPR.**

Asthma

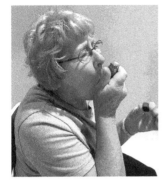

Asthma is a common condition where the airways go into spasm, causing tightness of the chest and severe difficulty breathing when someone is exposed to something that irritates their airways.

The airways become narrow; their lining becomes inflamed, starts to swell and can start producing sticky mucus or phlegm which makes it even harder to breath.

What causes asthma

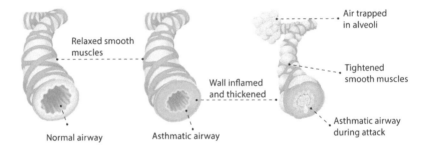

| Asthma and your airways

Elderly people often have complex breathing problems and anyone diagnosed with asthma should have their **blue reliever inhaler** within reach at all times.

1. Asthma can be triggered by all sorts of things:

- Exercise – this does not mean people should avoid exercise because they are asthmatic, but they should always have their blue reliever inhaler with them.
- Chemicals, smoke and fumes
- Cold air

- Colds and viruses
- Stress
- Household dust, fungi, moulds and pollen
- Specific allergens which can bring on a major asthma attack

Asthma sufferers will learn what their triggers are.

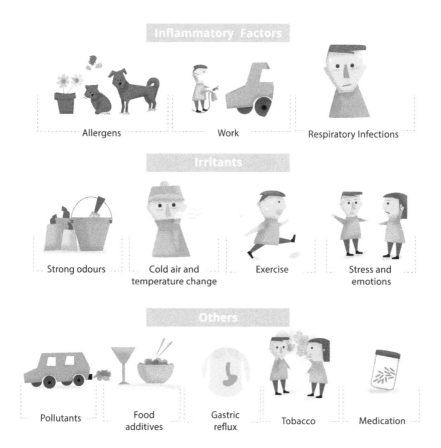

| Triggers for an asthma attack

2. Symptoms of asthma:

- Coughing

- Wheezing

- Shortness of breath

- Tightness in the chest

- Difficulty breathing out

- An increase in sticky mucus and phlegm

Asthmatics don't necessarily suffer from all these symptoms. Some people experience them from time to time; a few experience these symptoms all the time.

3. **Note:** encouraging someone to sit upright may be helpful when dealing with breathing problems. Sitting the wrong way on a chair may help.

Do **not** take them outside for fresh air if it is cold as cold air can make symptoms worse.

Spacers

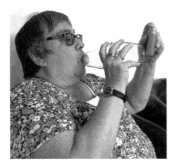

Using a spacer has been shown to deliver medication much more effectively, increasing the amount of medication reaching the airway, rather than hitting the back of the throat. This gives people much better control of their asthma.

There is a huge variety of shapes and sizes, but not all spacers fit all types of inhalers – use the spacer prescribed with the inhaler.

There is considerable co-ordination required to use an inhaler without a spacer and this can lead to increased stress and worsening of symptoms. Keep spacers with inhalers and have both available at all times.

How to use an inhaler

There are many different types of inhalers, these are some of the most common types:

The one you need if someone is having difficulty breathing is usually blue.

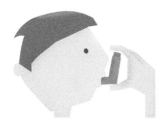

Standard inhaler technique: Remove the cap and shake the inhaler, breathe out, place the inhaler between your lips and inhale slowly and deeply at the same time as pressing to deliver the dose. Hold your breath for 10 seconds or as long as is comfortable. A second dose can be given in 30 seconds.

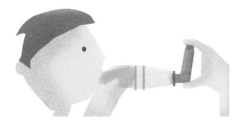

Using a Spacer improves the amount of medication reaching the lungs. Remove the cap from the inhaler, shake it and place into the end of the spacer. Breathe out gently and place the mouthpiece part of the spacer in the mouth, Press the inhaler once, breathe in and hold for 10 seconds or as long as is comfortable. A second dose can be given in 30 seconds.

For young children and some asthmatics they may use the multi-breath technique when they deliver a dose of medication and then breathe steadily 5 times in and out into the spacer. They should then remove the spacer from their mouth and repeat after 30 seconds if necessary.

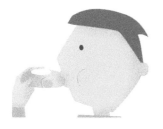

Inhaled dry powder inhalers need you to breathe out, close the mouth tightly around the mouthpiece and inhale rapidly to release the powder.

How to help in an asthma attack

Step 1

Help the casualty to take their usual dose of reliever (usually blue) inhaler immediately, preferably through a spacer.

Step 2

Sit the casualty upright
Get them to take slow steady breaths
Keep calm and try to keep them calm
Do not leave them unattended

Have the symptoms improved immediately?

No

Yes

Step 3

Continue to give two puffs of reliever inhaler every two minutes, up to 10 puffs

Continue to sit with the casualty until they are feeling completely well and can go back to previous activity

Step 4

If the casualty does not start to feel better after taking the reliever inhaler as above or if you are worried a any time call 999

Step 5

If an ambulance does not arrive within10 minutes repeat step 3 while you wait

Signs of an asthma attack can include any of these
Coughing
Being short of breath
Wheezy breathing
Being unusually quiet
Tightness in their chest

Follow the prescribed directions with the asthmatics medication. If the instructions are illegible or unavailable, use the following advice:

1. Be calm and reassuring. Reducing stress and keeping the casualty calm really helps them control their symptoms - panic can increase the severity of an attack.

2. Encourage the casualty to take one to two puffs of their reliever inhaler (usually blue), using a spacer if available.

3. Sit them down, loosen any tight clothing and encourage them to take slow, steady breaths.

4. If they do not start to feel better, they should take more puffs of their reliever inhaler; 2 every 2 minutes up to a maximum of 10 – or as prescribed.

5. If they do not start to feel better after taking the inhaler as above, or if you are worried, call 999.

6. Get them to keep taking their reliever inhaler whilst waiting for the paramedics.

People may have a variety of different asthma inhalers and medication to control their asthma – if they are having an asthma attack, it is the reliever inhaler that they need.

Reliever inhalers are usually blue, and these are the ones needed if they are short of breath and wheezing.

After an emergency asthma attack

Make an appointment with a doctor or asthma nurse for an asthma review within 48 hours of the attack.

Panic attacks and hyperventilation

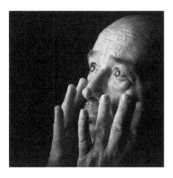

Most people have experienced a sense of panic at some time in their life - it is a perfectly normal response. Panic is an extreme feeling of fear and dread, and usually the overwhelming desire to escape an uncomfortable situation. Panic attacks can also occur suddenly with no obvious cause. Physical reactions may be frightening and can include the following:

- A pounding and racing heart or even palpitations (feeling your heart is stopping or missing beats)

- Shortness of breath or a feeling of choking

- Shaking, tingling or numbness in your fingers and toes

- Feeling sick and dizzy

- Sweating

- Needing the loo

- Thinking you might die

- Feeling you are losing control of your mind - even that you are going crazy

- Aggressiveness, sometimes shown through the wish to escape

1. Difficulty breathing due to panic attacks should not be confused with asthma. Asthma can be life-threatening - the casualty needs their medication and help quickly, whereas panic attacks are usually short lived, and the casualty quickly makes a full recovery.

   During asthma attacks, casualties usually wheeze as they struggle to breathe, whereas large volumes of air can be heard entering and leaving the lungs of a hyperventilating casualty.

If someone is having a panic attack

- Reassure them calmly; they may not be able to explain what has caused them to panic. Do not pressure them to do this, your supportive presence should help.

- Speak to them in positive, supportive terms – "you will be okay, this will pass in a minute" etc.

- Remove them from anything obvious that is causing distress.

- Encourage them to breathe calmly and slowly, in and out through their nose, to reduce the amount of carbon dioxide being lost.

- Small sips of water may help to calm them.

- If symptoms get worse, get medical help.

- When the panic attack is over, talk it through with them. Discuss relaxation techniques and other helpful means of coping in case this happens again.

2. Do **not** suggest breathing in and out of a paper bag. People used to think breathing in and out of a paper bag was helpful during a panic attack, and the physiology makes sense; breathing out in panic results in the loss of carbon dioxide in the blood, and breathing into a bag restores the lost CO_2.

   The danger with a paper bag is that the casualty becomes dependent upon it and can panic if they do not have one to hand. It is also extremely dangerous using a paper bag if someone is having an asthma attack and can make things worse.

   If attacks are persistent and severe, the patient can be referred for specialist help.

Allergic reactions and Anaphylactic shock

What is an allergic reaction?

Allergic reactions occur because the immune system reacts inappropriately to the presence of a substance it wrongly perceives as a threat. This can be touched, inhaled, swallowed or injected (during a routine vaccination or by an insect sting).

The body reacts to histamine released by cells damaged through the immune response.

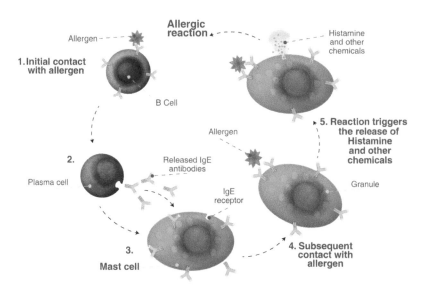

| *Allergic reaction diagram*

Everyone makes IgE, but people with allergies produce more of it. When someone with an allergic predisposition is exposed to an allergen, they produce a lot of IgE antibodies, that bind to the mast cells in the tissues or basophils in the blood. When the IgE line up next to each other, they affect the membranes of cells, causing them to break down (degranulation). The cells breaking down releases histamine and other chemicals. Histamine dilates blood vessels and makes them more permeable, so they lose fluid, causing swelling in the tissues.

Anaphylactic Reaction

This mechanism is so sensitive that minute quantities of an allergen can cause a reaction. The chemicals released act on blood vessels to cause swelling in the mouth and on the skin. There is a fall in blood pressure and in asthmatics the effect may be mainly on the lungs, causing a severe asthma attack which their inhaler is unable to help.

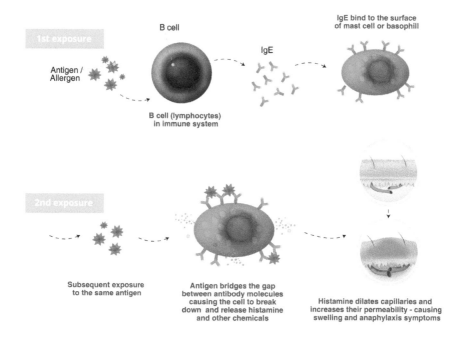

1st exposure

Antigen / Allergen

B cell

B cell (lymphocytes) in immune system

IgE

IgE bind to the surface of mast cell or basophill

2nd exposure

Subsequent exposure to the same antigen

Antigen bridges the gap between antibody molecules causing the cell to break down and release histamine and other chemicals

Histamine dilates capillaries and increases their permeabillty - causing swelling and anaphylaxis symptoms

Antihistamine can be effective for minor reactions

We have small amounts of histamine in our system normally, and we need it for various functions in the body - including regulating stomach acid and acting as a neurotransmitter in our nerve cells. However, larger amounts of histamine being released leads to symptoms such as sneezing, a blocked nose, itching etc. - the sort of symptoms often associated with hay fever and mild allergies. Antihistamine medication can work effectively at resolving these symptoms. However, Antihistamine medication typically takes around 15 minutes to work.

Anaphylaxis is life-threatening

Life-threatening and systemic allergic reactions are caused by the body producing extra histamine, which dilates small blood vessels and causes them to leak, resulting in swelling in areas such as the lungs, leading to breathing problems. Sufferers may have a rash and be flushed due to the increased blood supply to the skin. Their blood pressure may drop dramatically and they may collapse.

Frequency of exposure

The more times someone is exposed to a substance they react to, the quicker and more severe their reaction may become.

If they don't have a rash associated with the symptoms, it could still be an anaphylactic reaction; if they have a rapid onset of symptoms and may have been exposed to an allergen, treat it as an anaphylactic reaction.

Who is at risk from anaphylaxis?

Family history

It is thought that people inherit the predisposition to react to particular allergens, and this is combined with environmental factors. People can develop reactions to things that have never previously been a problem. If there is a family history, there is a far greater chance of someone having allergic tendencies.

Prone to severe reactions

If a patient has suffered a bad allergic reaction in the past – whatever the cause, this may make them more prone to having further severe reactions. If a significant reaction to a tiny dose occurs, or a reaction has occurred with just skin contact, this could indicate that they are sensitive to this particular allergen and greater contact could lead to a more severe attack.

Asthma higher risk

Asthma can put a patient at a higher risk during an allergic reaction and trigger an asthma attack that can't be resolved using their asthma pump. If someone is asthmatic and has an auto-injector, if they experience asthma type symptoms and their pump is not helping, they should use their adrenaline autoinjector immediately.

Allergens can be contained in some obscure products that you wouldn't automatically associate them with and so if someone appears to be having a reaction, with no obvious trigger, use their adrenaline auto-injector if indicated and get emergency help quickly.

Common triggers for reactions

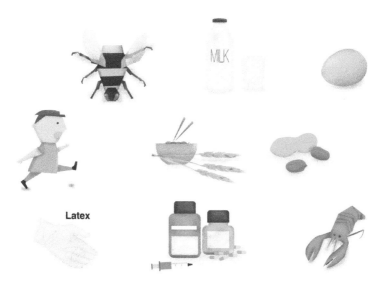

Individuals can react to absolutely anything.

Food triggers

The most common food triggers are peanuts, tree nuts (e.g. almonds, walnuts, cashews, and Brazil nuts), sesame seeds, fish, shellfish, dairy products and eggs.

Non-food triggers

Non-food causes include wasp or bee stings, natural latex (rubber), penicillin or any other drug or injection.

Exercise can also trigger a delayed allergic reaction following exposure to an allergen.

How to recognise an acute allergic reaction (anaphylactic shock)

A reaction can take many forms and people who have reacted one way when exposed to a particular allergen can react completely differently on another occasion when exposed to the same thing. It is therefore extremely difficult to predict what a reaction might look like.

Common symptoms

Flushed skin - General flushing of the skin

Rash or hives - A rash or hives anywhere on the body

Sense of impending doom – An overwhelming feeling of anxiety

Swelling of the throat - Swelling of the throat or mouth, causing difficulty swallowing or speaking

Heart rate - Alterations in heart rate – usually a speeding up of the heart

Asthma attack - Severe asthma attack which isn't relieved by their inhaler

Abdominal pain - Acute abdominal pain, violent nausea and vomiting

Feeling of weakness - A sudden feeling of weakness followed by collapse and unconsciousness

A patient is unlikely to experience all these symptoms.

How to Treat Anaphylaxis

1. The key advice is to avoid any known allergens.

2. If someone is having a mild allergic reaction, an antihistamine tablet or syrup can be very effective. However, the medication will take at least 15 minutes to work. If you are concerned that the reaction could be systemic (all over) and life-threatening, use an adrenaline auto-injector immediately. It is far better to give adrenaline unnecessarily than to give it too late.

3. Adrenaline auto-injectors are prescribed for those believed to be at risk. Adrenaline (also known as epinephrine) acts quickly, constricting blood vessels, relaxing the muscles in the lungs (improving breathing), stimulating the heartbeat and helping to stop swelling around the face and lips.

4. Acute allergic reactions can be life-threatening and it is crucially important you recognise the problem and know what to do quickly in order to save someone's life.

5. Adrenaline is the first choice for acute anaphylactic reaction and it works better the sooner it is given. Administer the injector, or help the sufferer administer it themselves, as quickly as possible and call for an ambulance stating clearly that the person is having an acute anaphylactic reaction.

6. Adrenaline should treat all the most dangerous symptoms of anaphylaxis rapidly, including throat swelling, difficulty breathing and low blood pressure. However, the casualty is likely to need additional medication in hospital to control their reaction.

7. Adrenaline is metabolised very quickly – it is very important that you call an ambulance as soon as an auto-injector has been given, as its effects can wear off within about 15 minutes. Another injector can be given 5-15 minutes after the first if necessary.

How to use an Adrenaline Auto-injector

There are currently 3 makes of Adrenaline Auto-injectors on the market in the UK; EpiPen, Jext and Emerade. They all contain adrenaline and are given in a similar manner. EpiPen is by far the most popular in the UK.

The adrenaline auto-injector should be carried at all times

If you have been prescribed an adrenaline auto-injector you should carry it with you at all times and register to receive a reminder when it is going out of date. If you have been prescribed 2 adrenaline injectors as a duo pack, you should carry both with you at all times in case a second dose is needed. Teach friends and family what to do if they need to help you or someone else having an anaphylactic reaction.

How to use

If you are giving an auto-injector to someone having an allergic reaction:

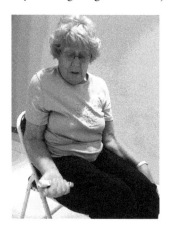

1. Hold the injector in your dominant hand, remove the safety cap with the other.

2. Put the injector firmly into the upper outer part of the casualty's thigh and hold it there for 3-10 seconds.

3. Remove it carefully and they should begin to feel better quite quickly.

4. If they continue to get worse, you may need to give another injector.

The auto-injector can be given through clothes.

Always phone an ambulance.

Patient positioning for anaphylaxis

Someone suffering from acute anaphylaxis is also likely to be showing signs of clinical shock.

Reassuring the casualty and positioning them appropriately can make a major difference to their recovery. They should also be kept warm and dry.

If someone is very short of breath, they should be encouraged to sit in an upright position to help their breathing. Put something under their knees to help increase their circulation. This is called the lazy-W position.

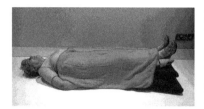 If they are not having difficulty breathing, but are feeling sick or dizzy and could be going into shock, they should lie down with their legs raised to help increase the circulation to their vital organs. Encourage them to turn their head to one side if they are likely to vomit. They should be covered to keep them warm and kept in this position until the paramedics arrive.

Do not get them up until they have been medically assessed.

Treat for shock by lying them down and raising their legs if they are showing symptoms of shock and are not having breathing problems.

After an anaphylactic reaction

An ambulance should always be called if someone is showing signs of anaphylaxis and they will usually be admitted overnight for observation. This is because some people have a second reaction some hours after the first.

Don't forget to replace used adrenaline auto-injectors.

Storage of auto-injectors

Easily accessible

Auto-injectors should be quickly and easily accessible and stored in a suitable container. Specifically designed containers are available from the relevant drug companies.

Clearly marked

The container should be clearly marked with its owner's name and include an instruction leaflet on how to use the injector. Personal treatment plans should be read by all relevant staff and be easily accessible should they be needed.

Store at room temperature

Auto-injectors should be stored at room temperature and kept away from direct sunlight.

Make sure you adhere to the expiry date – auto-injectors have a relatively short shelf life and once they have expired their adrenaline content diminishes. If auto-injectors are registered with the appropriate drug company, they will send automatic email or text alerts to warn you when the adrenaline injector is about to expire.

Legislation concerning the administration of adrenaline in a life-threatening emergency

"Medicines legislation restricts the administration of injectable medicines. Unless self-administered, they may only be administered by or in accordance with the instructions of a doctor (e.g. by a nurse). However, in the case of adrenaline there is an exemption to this restriction which means in an emergency, a suitably trained lay person is permitted to administer it by injection for the purpose of saving life. The use of an EpiPen to treat anaphylactic shock falls into this category.

Therefore, first aiders may administer an EpiPen if they are dealing with a life-threatening emergency in a casualty who has been prescribed and is in possession of an EpiPen and where the first aider is trained to use it."

25 January 2008 Health and Safety Executive Guidance

Wounds and bleeding

How to treat a bleeding wound

Wear gloves when dealing with bleeding. Dispose of soiled dressings in a yellow incinerator bag or in a sanitary bin.

If someone is bleeding, the priority is to **stop the blood coming out!** This seems completely logical, but when people are in the kitchen, they seem to automatically put wounds under the tap, losing their precious blood in the process!

It is never a priority to wash an injury – it will be cleaned in hospital if they need medical attention or can be cleaned later (after you have given immediate first aid) if you are dressing it yourself.

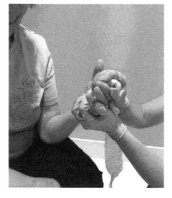

Sit or lie the casualty down – depending on the location and severity of the wound.

Examine the wound to see if there is anything embedded in it.

Pressure – apply direct pressure to stop the bleeding

Dress the wound

Shock due to bleeding

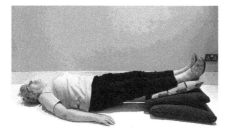

If the person is pale, cold, clammy (cold sweat) and showing signs of shock, or if there is a lot of blood, help their circulation by lying them down and raising their legs. Elevate the bleeding wound and apply direct pressure to control the bleeding.

Keep them warm and get emergency help.

Dressing

A dressing should be made of non-adherent, sterile material that will not stick to the wound, and be large enough to just cover the wound.

Applying a dressing

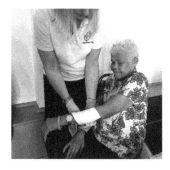

To apply a dressing, place a pad over the wound and firmly - but not too tightly - bandage over the top. Check you haven't put it on too tightly by squeezing the nail bed of the finger. The colour should come back as soon as you let go.

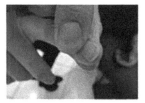 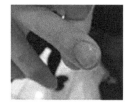

If blood comes through the first dressing, put another on top in the same way. If it comes through both, apply direct pressure with another cloth, elevate the wound and get medical help immediately. Be ready to treat for shock.

The purpose of a dressing

- To control bleeding
- To reduce the risk of shock
- To minimise risk of infection, both of the first aider and the casualty

Get appropriate medical attention quickly.

Embedded objects

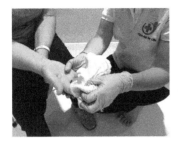

Never remove an embedded object from the wound. It will have caused damage on the way in and will damage again on the way out! It may also be stemming any bleeding.

The only exception is a small splinter that is clearly visible and easy to remove. If the splinter is on a joint, it should be removed by a health professional; it is possible the joint capsule has been damaged and this could lead to infection.

Apply pressure without pushing on the embedded object

Use a rolled cloth or triangular bandage to make a donut ring put this over the wound to enable you to apply pressure without pushing the embedded object further into the wound. Get medical help.

If you suspect that there is glass in the wound, the casualty will need an x-ray.

Removing a splinter

1. Clean the wound with warm soapy water

2. Use a pair of clean tweezers, grip the splinter close to the skin and gently pull it out at the same angle it appears to have entered.

3. Gently squeeze around the wound to encourage a little bleeding and ensure there is nothing remaining in the wound. Clean the wound once more, then cover it with a breathable sterile dressing.

4. Ensure the casualty's tetanus is up to date.

How much blood can you afford to lose?

The effect of blood loss

0.5 litres

Little or no effect on the body – equivalent to blood donation

Up to 2 litres

Adrenaline will be released which will speed up the pulse and cause sweating. The body starts to exhibit signs of shock.

2 litres

The pulse in the wrist can become undetectable as the body shuts down. Further blood loss will result in the casualty losing consciousness. The heart and breathing will eventually stop.

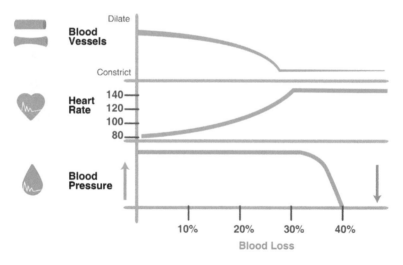

| *The effect of blood loss on the body*

Shock

Rapid pulse

Pale, cold and clammy

As shock develops:

The skin turns grey-blue and the lips tinged blue (cyanosis)

Weakness and dizziness

Nausea and vomiting

Thirst

Shallow, rapid breathing

As the brain is struggling for oxygen:

May become restless and possibly aggressive

A sense of 'impending doom'

Yawning and gasping for air

Eventually they will lose consciousness, become unresponsive and finally stop breathing

Symptoms of shock

Shock is 'a lack of oxygen to the tissues of the body, usually caused by a fall in blood volume or blood pressure'.

Shock occurs as a result of the body's circulatory system failing to work properly. It means the tissues and organs of the body - including the heart and the brain - struggle to get sufficient oxygen. The body's response is to shut down circulation to the skin. This means the casualty becomes pale, cold and clammy (with cold, wet skin). The heart speeds up as it tries to get sufficient blood supply and oxygen around the body, and blood supply is drawn away from the gut to prioritise vital organs. This makes the casualty feel sick and thirsty. They may also feel anxious, dizzy and a bit confused as their brain suffers from lack of oxygenated blood. If shock is untreated it can be fatal.

Shock results from major drop in blood pressure and is serious; it should not be confused with the frightened reaction people have when faced with a scary situation. It is often clinical shock that results in people dying from an acute injury or illness.

The most common types of shock

Hypovolaemic – The body loses fluid, such as with major bleeds (internal and external), burns, diarrhoea and vomiting

Cardiogenic – i.e. heart attack; the heart is not pumping effectively

Anaphylactic – The body reacts to something releasing large amounts of Histamine and other hormones. These dilate the blood vessels and means they leak fluid, causing swelling of the airways and leading to a triple whammy of shock.

Extremes of temperature can also cause the body to go into shock, as can a major assault on the nervous system such as a spinal or brain injury.

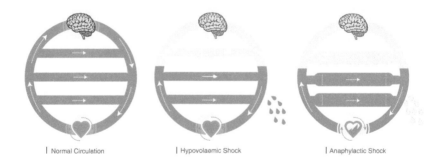

| Normal Circulation | Hypovolaemic Shock | Anaphylactic Shock

Treatment of shock

If shock is due to a major bleed

If the shock is due to a major bleed, apply pressure to the wound and get them to lie down and raise their legs.

If shock is due to a heart attack

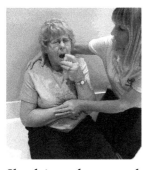

If you suspect the shock is caused by a heart attack, put them in the lazy-W position. If they have a severe head injury or you are worried about their spine, keep them still, support their head and neck and avoid them twisting their spine.

Reassure them and keep them warm

Cover them to keep them warm.

Shock is made worse when someone is cold, anxious or in pain. Reassuring and keeping them warm can make a real difference.

Call an ambulance

Moisten their lips if they are complaining of thirst – do not give them a drink. They may need an operation and it is safer to give someone a general anaesthetic when they have an empty stomach.

Internal bleeding

Internal bleeding can be difficult to diagnose. The body can lose large amounts of blood from a ruptured organ, major fracture or stabbing, which on the surface does not look too serious.

Key Signs of Internal Bleeding

The key signs and symptoms of internal bleeding are those of shock

- Pale, cold, clammy, feeling sick and thirsty

- Possible bruising

- Chest pain

- Abdominal pain

- Swelling in the affected area

- Seepage from orifices – this may be discovered by the casualty or later in a medical environment. A first aider should not be looking for blood loss in any intimate areas.

  Call an ambulance

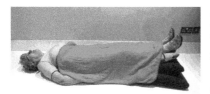
If they show signs of shock, position them in the best way to increase blood flow to the heart and brain – this is usually lying down with their legs raised. Cover them with a blanket.

Amputated parts

Amputating the tip of a finger or toe is a common injury experienced by older people, however, with the right initial first aid treatment, they can very often be successfully re-attached.

If part of the finger (or toe) is amputated

If part of a finger is amputated, the priority is to look after the casualty.

- Sit them down, reassure them and grab a cloth to apply direct pressure to the stump

- Elevate the injured hand above the level of the heart. Do not worry about the amputated part until bleeding has been controlled and the casualty is calmer.

  Save the amputated part

Pick up the finger. Do **not** wash it.

Wrap it in a cloth, put this in a plastic bag and put that on an ice pack.

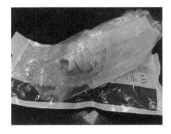

Do not let the ice come directly into contact with the amputated part; this could cause ice burns and mean the finger will not be able to be sewn back. You are chilling, not freezing the amputated part to prevent it decomposing. Transport the casualty and amputated finger to hospital, if necessary by ambulance.

Partially attached

If the finger is still partly attached, with a blood supply, bandage the severed part carefully in situ, not too tightly. Support and elevate the hand and get emergency medical help.

Crushed and bruised fingers

If fingers are crushed and bruised, but no bits are missing, hold the injured area under cool running water for 10 minutes, then apply a wrapped ice pack. Elevate the injured hand and seek medical advice.

Wear gloves when dealing with bleeding.

Knocked out teeth

A whole tooth that has been knocked out can be kept alive and re-implanted.

If someone falls and their tooth is knocked out, complete with its root, advise the person to bite on a clean cloth to stem the bleeding. Apply a wrapped ice pack to reduce the swelling to their face. Pick up the tooth and put it in milk or saliva to keep it alive. Transport the casualty and their tooth to a good dentist or a dental hospital and the tooth may be able to be re-implanted.

Eye injuries

Eye injuries can be very unpleasant and painful. If someone has grit or dust in their eye, rinse it out with water.

Something embedded in eye

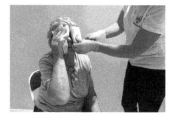

If something is embedded in the eye, get the casualty to cover both eyes as moving one will result in the other moving too. Do not attempt to remove anything embedded in the eye.

Cuts to the eyelid

If someone has a cut to their eyelid, do not apply pressure. The best thing to do is to get a clean compress and then cover the eye with a small paper cup to prevent bacteria or debris getting into the cut and get medical help.

Chemicals in the eye

If someone gets chemicals in their eye, wash it immediately with cold water or a saline eye wash and transport the person to hospital.

1. Wear gloves.
2. Rinse the casualty's eye with cool running water for at least 10 minutes.
3. Cover the affected eye with a non-fluffy pad if necessary.
4. Transfer to a hospital ideally with a specialist eye department.
5. Take details of the chemicals with you to the hospital.
    If the chemicals have made the person sensitive to light, cover their head with a towel before taking them to the hospital.

Nose bleeds

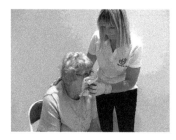

Nose bleeds are remarkably common. Small children often get nose bleeds as they have small blood vessels in their noses, which dilate and burst when they get warm. The same can happen with older people as their blood vessels become thinner. Nose bleeds can also be an indicator of high blood pressure.

What to do

- Encourage them to sit down.

- Grab something to catch the blood

- Lean the casualty forward, pinching the bridge of their nose. Doing this will allow you to see when the bleeding has stopped and prevent blood trickling down the back of their throat which could make them sick.

- Apply pressure externally on the nose to try and push the leaking blood vessel against the inside of the nose to compress it and stop it bleeding.

- Keep changing your grip until you have got to a point where no blood is coming out.

- Keep applying pressure for at least 10 minutes.

- Release pressure slightly and if it starts to bleed again, hold for another 10 minutes. Repeat this step if necessary.

If it won't stop

If it really won't stop bleeding, you will need medical help. Advise them not to pick, poke or blow their nose.

Special situation

If the nose bleed has been caused by trauma, you may not be able to stop the bleeding. You need to apply pressure to try and reduce the amount of blood coming out as loss of blood is dangerous. Apply a wrapped ice pack, keep applying pressure and get medical help.

Varicose veins

It is common for older people to have varicose veins. These are engorged veins that commonly occur on the back of the legs and result from faulty valves and weakened vessels. If these veins are injured by something like a shopping trolley, wheelchair or buggy accidently being driven into them, they will bleed profusely. It is vital to apply pressure urgently to stop the bleeding. Lie them down, raise their legs and apply firm pressure. Call for an ambulance immediately.

Types of wounds

Grazes

Grazes are superficial injuries caused by some of the skin being scraped off to reveal a dirty wound. It is never a priority to clean the wound immediately. Usually it can be patched up with a plaster and cleaned properly a short time later, in an environment where you can wash your hands, wear gloves and use gauze and water or sterile wipes to clean it thoroughly.

Cleaning

1. Clean the worst of the dirt from around the wound with a cloth.

2. Using sterile gauze and clean water, or an antiseptic wipe, clean from the inside of the wound outwards in one sweep.

3. Throw the gauze away and use a new sterile piece to wipe from the inside outwards again. Discard this and use another piece until the wound is completely clean and devoid of any dirt or grit.

A dirty wound will not heal and is likely to become infected.

Apply a non-adherent dressing pad, shiny side down onto the wound and secure with some tape or a dressing with a bandage.

Remove the dressing at night to allow air to get to the wound. Avoid soaking in a bath or going swimming until the wound has healed properly.

Any soiled dressings or gauze should be disposed of in an incinerator bin – either given to the emergency services to dispose of, or put into a sanitary bin.

The casualty should be encouraged to check their tetanus status.

Incised wound

An incised wound is a clean edged wound created by a sharp object.

Laceration

This sort of wound involves a lot of tissue damage and often crushing or ripping of the body. It can look very frightening, but the treatment is the same as for any other wound.

Puncture wounds

Often caused by a sharp object with a deep track of internal damage, contamination and germs. There may be a small entry wound but a lot of internal damage. A stab wound can be a type of puncture wound. Never remove an object left in a wound.

Contusion

Another word for a bruise, which is bleeding under the skin. Apply a wrapped ice pack for 10 minutes to reduce bruising.

Fainting

Fainting is a brief loss of consciousness, caused by a temporary reduction in the blood flow of the brain.

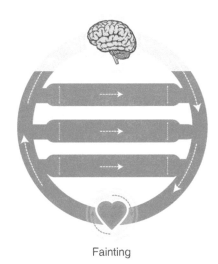

Fainting

Fainting can be a reaction to pain, lack of food, exhaustion or emotional stress. People often feel faint because it is warm, or they have been exercising and then stop; the small blood vessels in their skin become dilated and blood begins to pool in their feet. Lying down with raised legs will improve circulation and redirect blood to the brain. This should make the casualty feel better or come around quickly. If they don't, you will need to put them into the recovery position.

Bites and Stings

Bee Stings

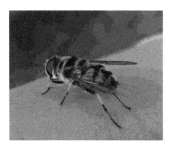

If someone has been stung by a bee and the sting is still in the skin, quickly flick it out using your thumb nail or a credit card. It is important not to squeeze the sting as this can increase the amount of allergen entering the body and amplify any potential allergic reaction. Wasps and other stinging insects do not leave the sting behind in the wound.

If the casualty has a local reaction, apply a wrapped ice pack to reduce swelling. Piriton (Chlorphenamine antihistamine) is also helpful. Oral Antihistamine takes about 15 minutes to work.

If the casualty shows any signs of having a systemic reaction or of anaphylactic shock, call an ambulance immediately and use their Adrenaline Auto-injector if they have one. Reassuring them and positioning them appropriately can make a major difference to their treatment. They should also be kept warm and dry.

Giving an adrenaline auto-injector

If someone is very short of breath, they should be encouraged to sit in an upright position to help their breathing, putting something under their knees to help increase circulation. This is the lazy-W position.

If they are not having difficulty breathing, but are pale, cold, clammy and feeling sick or thirsty, they should lie down with their legs raised to help increase circulation to their vital organs. Encourage them to turn their head to one side if they are likely to vomit. They should be covered to keep them warm and kept in this position until the paramedics arrive.

Animal bites

Bites from animals can be jagged and often get infected. Even if an animal bite has just punctured the skin, it is important to wash the wound really well and look out for any sign of infection. It is sensible to get any bite that has punctured the skin looked at by a medical professional. If the wound looks red and becomes inflamed, hot, or angry-looking, it is getting infected and the casualty will need antibiotics.

Treating the bite

The initial treatment for a bite is the same as for any other wound, except it is important to wash it immediately with clean water and antibacterial soap (depending where the person has been bitten).

1. Reassure the casualty
2. Wash the wound thoroughly with clean water (and antibacterial soap depending on the location of the wound)
3. Elevate the wound and apply pressure to stop bleeding
4. Be ready to treat for shock.

Note: outside the UK, if someone is bitten or licked in a wound, it is really important to get medical attention quickly and have anti-rabies medication. It is also important to ensure that they are covered for tetanus.

Burns

What to do with a burn

Treat all burns immediately with cool running water.

1. Immediately, but extremely carefully, remove loose clothing covering the burn. Do not take clothes off if there is any risk the skin has stuck to them or it has blistered.
2. Put the affected area under cool running water for at least 10 minutes. Remember you are cooling the burn, not the casualty.
3. Keep them warm and dry and be aware for any signs of shock.

When to phone for an ambulance

Phone an ambulance if a large area is affected, or the skin is broken or blistered. Keep the area under cool running water while you wait for the ambulance.

Assessing the severity of a burn

Size

Cause

Age

Location

Depth

Size – the larger the area involved, the more serious it is for the casualty and the more likely they are to suffer from shock. A burn is measured using the size of your hand – 1 hand is 1% of your body.

Cause – How the burn was caused can affect on-going treatment.

Age – Burns are more serious in babies, children and the elderly.

Location – Where on the body is the burn located. Burns to the hands, face, feet, genitals, airway, or a burn that extends all the way around a limb, are particularly serious.

Depth – How deep is the burn; superficial, partial-thickness or full-thickness?

Causes of burns

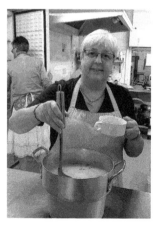

- Steam
- Flames
- Hot liquids (this is called a scald)
- Friction
- Hot objects such as irons, electric hobs or heated towel rails
- Ice and extremely cold objects
- Chemicals
- Radiation – sun lamps

If the burn is caused by a chemical, run it under cool running water for at least 20 minutes and be careful of its run-off as it could still be corrosive and hurt you. Look at the advice on its packaging and see if there are any specific instructions.

Sunburn

Prevent sunburn by avoiding the main heat of the day, wearing sun cream, hats and sun-resistant material.

If someone is sunburnt

1. Cool the area under a shower for at least 10 minutes, or repeatedly apply cool wet towels for 15 minutes.

2. When completely cooled, apply neat Aloe Vera gel to the affected area. This will soothe, reduce swelling and promote healing.

3. Give the casualty plenty to drink and seek medical advice

Electrical burns

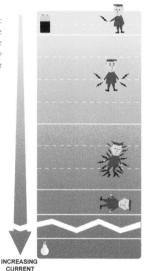

Effects can range from a tingle to cardiac arrest. There is no exact way to predict the injury from any given amperage. The table below shows generally how degree of injury relates to current passing through a body for a few seconds.

The effect of electric shock on the human body is determined by three main factors:

1 How much current is flowing through the body (measured in amperes and determined by voltage and resistance).

2 The path of current through the body.

3 How long the body is in the circuit.

INCREASING
CURRENT

Mild Shock
Trip setting for ground fault circuit interrupter

Muscle Contractions
Victim cannot let go

Severe Shock
Breathing difficult - possible respiratory arrest

Heart Stops pumping

Increasing probability of death

Enough current to light a 100 - watt bulb

| *Electric shock*

Always ensure the environment is safe if someone has been electrocuted. Do not touch them until you have turned the electricity off at the mains. Electrical burns have an entry and exit and burn all the way through the inside. Therefore, the electrical burn is unlikely to be the most important injury and should not be a distraction. They may be losing consciousness and could stop breathing as a result of the shock affecting their heart.

All burns are serious; particularly so when it is a child or someone elderly that is burnt. People often have different depths of burn within a single injury. Whatever the depth of burn, they should all be treated under cool running water.

Determine the depth of the burn

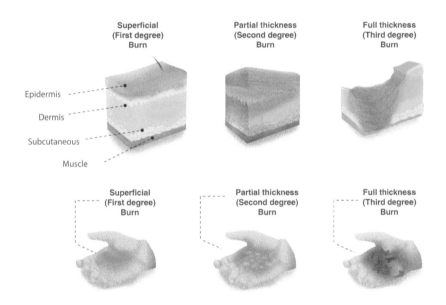

A **superficial** burn only affects the top layer of skin. It is really painful and likely to blister.

A **partial thickness** burn is painful. The burn has gone through both the first and second layer of skin.

Full thickness burns are often not as painful as the nerves have been very severely damaged too. This is the most severe sort of burn; the skin may appear pale, white or charred it will require extensive treatment and skin grafts.

Treating a burn

Treating a burn promptly makes a huge difference to its severity and therefore the amount of pain, scarring and length of time in hospital the casualty suffers.

Never touch the burn, pop blisters, or put any cream on it. Take burns very seriously and always seek medical advice.

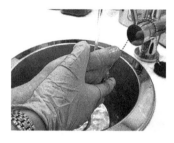

Cool the burn under cool running water (keep the casualty warm).

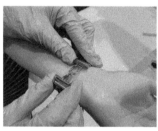

Remove any watches, jewellery etc. and loose clothing.

Dressing a burn

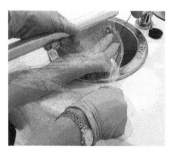

A burn can be dressed using clean clingfilm, loosely applied. Discard the first couple of turns of cling film and place an inner piece loosely over the burn. A burn should never be dressed until it has been cooled for at least 15 minutes. Covering a burn reduces the risk of infection and reduce pain by covering exposed nerve endings. If the burn is large enough to require **dressing,** phone for an ambulance and keep cooling the burn under cool running water. The paramedics will dress it for you.

Always get a medical professional to assess a burn.

Never

- Remove anything that has stuck to a burn
- Touch a burn
- Burst blisters
- Apply any creams, lotions or fats
- Apply tight dressings, tapes or use anything fluffy

Inhalation of fumes

Take the casualty away from smoke and fumes and encourage them to breathe fresh air if possible. Check consciousness, airway and breathing and be prepared to resuscitate if necessary. Burns to the airway must be treated as an **urgent medical emergency.**

Smoke inhalation can cause difficulty breathing, blueness around the lips, they may have soot around their mouth and could have a hoarse voice and painful throat. If they are fully conscious, sitting them upright to help their breathing and giving small sips of cool water is helpful. Do not leave them; continually reassess them to ensure they are not losing consciousness.

Carbon Monoxide is a silent killer as there is no smell or smoke associated with it.

Poisoning

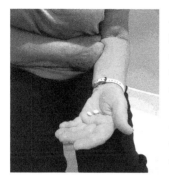

A poison is any substance (a solid, liquid, or a gas) which can cause damage if it enters the body in sufficient quantities. A poison can be swallowed, breathed in, absorbed through the skin or injected.

Some poisons cause an all-over reaction; this can result in seizures, blurred vision, acute anaphylaxis or be fatal.

If you suspect someone has taken a harmful substance, call an ambulance and explain clearly what has happened. They will advise you what to do.

Prevention

- Be mindful about substances
- Fit carbon monoxide alarms and have them and all appliances checked regularly
- Use original containers

Never decant medication into different containers; always use the original, clearly labelled. If the label has worn off and you are no longer sure what was in it, dispose of it carefully.

However, specially designed pill organisers can be extremely helpful for remembering when and how to take medication.

Make sure people needing to take numerous pills are competent with their medication. If necessary pharmacists can help by supplying pre-prepared pill boxes to make it easier for people to take the right medication at the prescribed times.

Poisoning from an ingested substance

If you find someone occupied with their pills or any other potentially poisonous substance, and are unsure if they have taken anything, always get them checked!

Depending what they have taken, they may have a burning sensation of the lips and mouth, nausea or vomiting, drowsiness or hyper-mania and possibly a change in their heartbeat.

If someone has swallowed a non-corrosive substance (a product that will not burn them) and seems completely well:

1. Encourage them to stay calm and still

Moving around will increase their metabolism and speed up the poison circulating around the body.

2. Try not to be cross or angry with them

They will not tell you what they have taken if they are scared or feel uncomfortable.

3. Phone 111 or the poisons unit and get advice from them

If they become unconscious

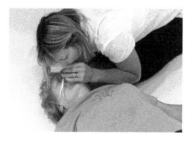

If the casualty becomes unconscious, open the airway and check for breathing. Be ready to resuscitate if necessary. Use a protective face shield to ensure you don't put yourself at risk from whatever they have ingested.

Tip: If someone has swallowed a berry from a plant, take a photo of the plant and a leaf as well. These will help the medical team to identify the berry and establish whether it is harmful or not.

Falls

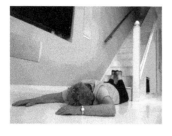

Falls are a major cause of older people needing to be admitted to hospital and it can have a major impact on their confidence and future mobility. Older people frequently fracture their hips due a fall and this may result in them losing their independence and needing to be cared for.

- If someone gets muddled and confused, they can be at greater risk of injuring themselves.

- Home hazards are frequently a cause of accidents; loose stair carpets, rugs, poorly-fitting footwear and slippers that no longer have sufficient grip.

- Most older people's eyesight gets weaker and they can struggle particularly in low light; failing to see the top step of the stairs or tripping over things left in hazardous places. As people get older it can be helpful to have a distinct change of colour to highlight the step at the top of the stairs or other potential hazards.

- Medication to reduce high blood pressure can result in dizziness from getting up too quickly. This can lead to wobbling and potentially to collapse. Anyone on blood pressure reducing tablets should be encouraged to get up very slowly, while holding onto something.

Incontinence or urgency for the toilet

People are more likely to have accidents if they have problems with incontinence. If they are desperate to go to the toilet they may rush, resulting in them falling, and if they have not made it in time they can end up slipping on a wet floor.

Carers should consider all these risks and work with the person they are caring for as well as any external organizations to assess the likelihood of falling and minimise the risks.

If you have had a fall:

Stay as calm as you can. Don't rush to get up; take time to establish whether you are hurt. Lie still and work systematically up your body to check for pain or bleeding when moving your limbs. If you feel able to get yourself up, do this slowly. Roll onto your hands and knees and look for a stable piece of furniture, such as a chair or bed. Hold onto this with both hands and use it to help get yourself up (see detailed instructions *The best way to get up after a fall*). Take time to rest and contact someone to let them know what has happened.

If you're hurt or unable to get up, try to get someone's attention by calling for help. Use your mobile phone if you have one to hand, otherwise bang on the wall or floor to alert neighbours, or press your emergency aid call button, if you have one. Alternatively, try and crawl to your telephone and call someone local or dial 999 to call an ambulance.

Do not exhaust yourself trying to get help. Remain calm and if possible cover yourself with something warm, such as a rug or coat. Wrap yourself up as well as you can and get as comfortable as possible. It is important to shift your body weight frequently to prevent pressure sores.

The best way to get up after a fall:

- Lie still for a couple of minutes and check you really are not hurt. Work systematically up your body to check for pain or bleeding when moving your limbs.

- If you feel able to get yourself up, do this slowly. Roll onto your hands and knees and look for a stable piece of furniture, such as a chair or bed. Find something soft to kneel on to protect your knees.

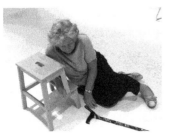

Hold on to the furniture with both hands and use the furniture to assist you in getting up.

Take time to rest and contact someone to tell them what has happened.

Look for something sturdy to pull yourself up onto and crawl or manoeuvre yourself over to it.

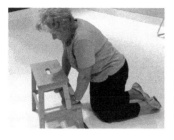

Move onto your knees – put padding under your knees if necessary and stabilise yourself onto the chair or stable piece of furniture that you are going to use to get yourself up.

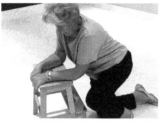

Bend up one leg and plant your foot firmly on the ground. Use the chair or furniture to carefully push yourself up. Take your time.

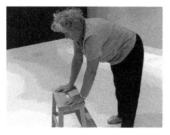

Remain supported with your head forward until you are sure you have properly got your balance. Carefully push yourself up to a standing position.

Get any grazes or cuts checked by a medical professional. Particularly on shins as it is important that they are appropriately assessed, cleaned and dressed to avoid leg ulcers.

Breaks, Sprains and Dislocations

Is it a broken a bone?

The honest answer is, unless the bone is sticking out, or the limb is at a very peculiar angle, the only way to know for sure that a bone is broken is to have an x-ray.

A fracture is another word for a broken bone.

Other possible symptoms:

Pain – it hurts

Loss of power – it can be hard to move a broken limb

Unnatural movement – the limb may be at an odd angle and have a wider range of movement than it should have

Swelling – bruising or a wound around the fracture site

Deformity – limbs may be shortened, or the broken area could have lumps and bumps or stepping (with an injured spine it is uneven as you gently feel down their back)

Irregularity – lumps, bumps, depressions or stretched skin

Crepitus – the grinding sound when the end of bones rub against each other

Tenderness – pain at the site of injury

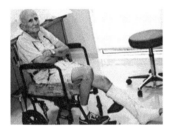

Broken bones on their own rarely cause fatalities. However, if there is bleeding associated with the injury (either internal or external) this can cause the casualty to go into shock, which is life-threatening. Keep the casualty warm and dry and be aware that pain and stress will adversely affect their condition.

If you are at all worried about someone you think may have broken a bone, phone an ambulance.

Types of Fractures

Open fractures

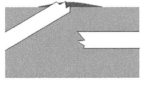

Open Fracture

If the bone is sticking out, it is broken! Your priority is to **stop bleeding,** without pushing on the bone or moving the broken limb at all. Then get emergency help.

Be very aware of the onset of shock – keep them warm and dry. If they show any signs of shock, lie them down, but do not elevate their legs if either one is broken.

Complicated fractures

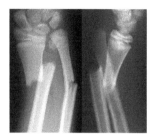

With complicated fractures, muscles, nerves, tendons and blood vessels could be trapped and damaged. If someone has lost feeling in part of their limb, or it has changed colour, they will need urgent medical treatment.

Keep them calm and warm.

Closed fractures

With a closed fracture, the bone has not come through the skin.

PRICE: Treatment for soft tissue injuries and closed fractures

Protect the injury (stop using the injured limb, pad to protect)

Rest the injury

Ice – apply a wrapped ice pack

Comfortable support – apply a supportive bandage

Elevate – to reduce swelling

When to call an ambulance

Call an ambulance if you are worried in any way, or if:
- They start to show signs of shock
- There is a possibility they have injured their spine or head
- They have any difficulty breathing or begin to lose consciousness
- It is an open fracture, with the bone through the skin
- They lose feeling in the limb, or it changes colour dramatically

- You are unable to safely transport the casualty to hospital yourself, keeping the limb stable and supported
- There is a suspected pelvic or hip fracture
- You are worried about them in any way.

Dislocation

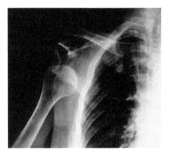

A dislocation occurs when a bone is pulled out of position at a joint and it can be accompanied by other tissue damage.

Always get a medical professional to put a dislocated joint back as you could cause further damage and trap nerves or blood vessels trying to put it back yourself.

Signs of dislocation

- Difficulty moving the joint, pain and stiffness
- Swelling and bruising around the joint
- Asymmetry, with one joint looking deformed and out of place
- A shortening, bending or twisting of the joint

Treatment

Support the injury to avoid unnecessary and painful movement (the casualty may prefer to do this themselves)

- Never try and reposition the limb yourself
- Look out for signs of shock
- Transport them to hospital or phone an ambulance
- Do not allow them to eat or drink as they may need a general anaesthetic

If someone has dislocated their jaw, do not bandage it as this could be very dangerous – get them to support their lower jaw by cupping it in their hands and get them to hospital.

Slings

Broad arm sling to support a sprained wrist

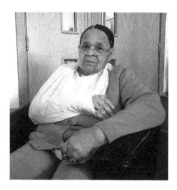

1. Use a triangular bandage. Put it under the injured arm with the 90° corner on the elbow.

2. Slip it under the injured arm to support it and wrap it over the top, securing the sling on the neck.

3. Tie a knot to fasten the sling.

4. Secure the corner by twisting and tucking in, or use a safety pin or tape.

Note: casualties often prefer to support their injury themselves than have a sling.

Head injuries

As people get older they are more likely to fall and knock their head. It can be difficult to tell whether a head injury is serious or not.

Fortunately, most falls or blows to the head result in injury to the scalp only, which can be very frightening (the head and face are very vascular so injuries bleed profusely) but not life-threatening. However, severe or repeated head injuries can result in damage to the brain. An internal head injury may become apparent immediately, or up to a couple of days after the accident. Someone who has sustained a head injury should ideally not be on their own for the next 48 hours and refrain from driving until they have been fully assessed. If anything unusual is observed, seek medical attention immediately (see section below on signs of compression). If you are in any doubt, get medical attention – they will do a CT scan in hospital to establish the extent of the injury if they are concerned.

What to do

Call an ambulance if a casualty complains of head and neck pain or isn't walking normally following a head injury.

If the casualty is alert and behaving normally after the fall or blow:

- Talk to the casualty to check that they are fully alert and orientated; that they know where they are and what happened.

- Apply a wrapped ice pack or instant cold pack to the injured area for 10 minutes.

- Observe them carefully for the next 48 hours. If you notice anything unusual, phone an ambulance immediately.

Suspected brain injury

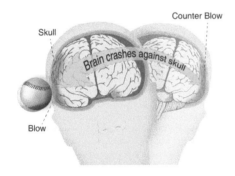

Counter Blow

Skull

Brain crashes against skull

Blow

Remember a serious head injury can also result in a spinal injury due to the whiplash effect.

The brain is cushioned by cerebrospinal fluid; a severe blow to the head may knock the brain into the side of the skull or tear blood vessels, like a jelly in a box. Any internal head injury — fractured skull, torn blood vessels, or damage to the brain itself — can cause the brain to swell. This can be serious and potentially life-threatening. Different levels of injury require different levels of concern. It can be difficult to determine the level of injury, so it's always wise to discuss a head injury with your doctor. A clear indicator of a more serious injury is when someone loses consciousness or is confused.

Signs and symptoms to look out for following a head injury

The following signs and symptoms can appear immediately or over the next couple of days. Keep a close eye on the casualty and get medical advice if at all concerned.

Experienced by Casualty

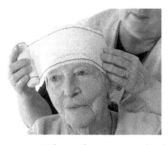

- Headache or pressure in the head
- Balance problems or dizziness
- Nausea/vomiting
- Sensitivity to light or noise
- Does not feel right
- Blurred vision or double vision
- Feel "dazed", sluggish, foggy or groggy
- Difficulty concentrating or remembering
- Feeling irritable, sad, nervous or more emotional
- Sleep disturbances

Observed by others

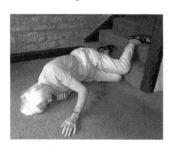

- Appears stunned or dazed
- Loses consciousness (even briefly)
- Is confused about events
- Trouble thinking or concentrating
- Can't recall events prior or after event
- Shows behaviour or personality changes
- Answer questions slowly and repeats questions
- Has difficulty remembering things and organising themselves

Compression and concussion

If the brain is injured it will swell and may bleed, in the same way as any other injury. The difference is, if the brain swells, it can only press against other parts of the brain and the spinal cord. This results in compression of these vital organs and can be fatal. Compression can happen almost immediately, or up to 48 hours after the bang on the head and even longer if they bang their head again.

Concussion

Concussion is a reversible form of brain injury. Following a bad bang on the head, a casualty may be in pain, have short-term loss of memory, feel dizzy and be confused. Someone with concussion should always be monitored for signs of compression. If you see anything unusual at all, phone for an ambulance. Do not leave anyone who has had a severe head injury on their own – they should have someone else with them to look out for signs of brain injury.

Compression

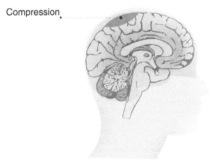

|Cerebral compression

When to call an ambulance

- Unconsciousness
- Abnormal breathing
- Obvious serious wound or suspected skull fracture
- Bleeding or clear fluid from the nose, ear or mouth

- Lack of co-ordination
- Disturbance of speech or vision
- Pupils of unequal size
- Weakness or paralysis
- Dizziness
- Neck pain or stiffness
- Fitting
- Vomiting

If the casualty is unconscious:

- If they are breathing, roll them into the recovery position (on their side so that their tongue falls forward in their mouth and any vomit can drain away), trying not to twist their neck or spine at all. Any head injury may well have caused spinal damage as the head recoils from the blow.
- If they are not breathing start CPR.
- Call for an ambulance.

If the casualty is conscious and it is a serious head injury:

- Phone for an ambulance
- Do your best to keep the casualty calm and still – make sure they do not twist, as they could have a spinal injury.
- If there is bleeding, grab a clean cloth and apply pressure.
- Do **not** attempt to clean the wound as it could make things worse.
- Do **not** apply forceful direct pressure to the wound if you suspect the skull is fractured.
- Do **not** remove any object that's stuck in the wound.

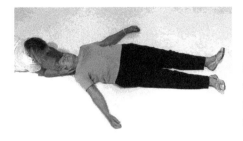

Support their head and neck without covering their ears to keep their spine in line and encourage them not to twist.

Skull Fracture

Signs:

- Watery blood coming from their ear, nose or head
- Bruising around their eyes or behind an ear
- An open wound on the head

If they are conscious

- Keep them as still as you can, don't let them twist as they could well have a spinal injury
- Get the emergency services on their way immediately

If they are unresponsive and breathing normally

- Put them in the recovery position
- Protect their spine and do your best not to let them twist
- If they are unconscious and not breathing, start CPR

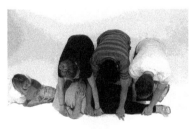 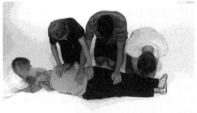

Support their head and neck, without covering their ears. Carefully roll them into the recovery position keeping their spine straight. Keep supporting their head and neck – do not let go until the paramedics are able to take over.

Special consideration

If you are looking after a casualty who is unresponsive and breathing, and are worried about the possibility of a spinal injury; **if you have been trained to recognise the early signs of airway obstruction and are confident in doing so**, keep the casualty in the position that they have landed and support their head and neck using MILS (Manual In-Line Stabilisation). Get someone to phone an ambulance immediately.

If you are at all concerned about their airway, put them into the recovery position immediately. Keep monitoring their breathing.

Strokes and Trans-Ischaemic Attacks (TIAs)

A stroke is a disturbance to the blood flow of the brain caused by a blockage or bleed in one of the blood vessels supplying the brain. Blockages to the brain are a lot more common than bleeds. Both have the same symptoms.

What you are looking for

- **Face** – can they smile and show their teeth?
- **Arms** – can they raise their arms and keep them held there, or does one arm fall?
- **Speech** – can they repeat a phrase you give them? Is their speech slurred? Do they have difficulty remembering words?
- **Tongue** - if they stick their tongue out is it crooked to one side or another?
- Unequal pupils

What causes a stroke

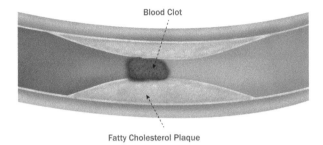

A stroke is caused either by a bleed or by a build-up of plaque and fatty deposits in the arteries (like angina and heart attacks). When these plaques break away, or if they slow the blood flow to the extent that it forms a clot, they can block a blood vessel supplying the brain and cause a stroke.

A Trans-Ischaemic Attack (TIA) can cause stroke-like symptoms that go away fairly quickly. The arteries in the brain have become blocked by fatty plaques (in the same way as with angina in the heart) and TIAs are warning signs that someone is at high risk of having a stroke. Any stroke-like symptoms should be taken seriously and a medical professional consulted immediately. Early diagnosis and treatment can prevent a full stroke.

If someone is showing the signs of a stroke, phone an ambulance immediately and get them to a specialist Stroke Unit as soon as possible. **Time is really important** – if the stroke is caused by a blood clot and they are able to receive clot-busting drug treatment (Alteplase) within 3 hours, the symptoms of the stroke can often be reversed.

Spinal injury

Consider a spinal injury if:

- Someone has fallen a distance more than twice their height

- Someone has been pushed with force

- Something heavy has fallen onto them

- They have been involved in a road traffic accident – either within a moving vehicle or being hit by anything at speed, particularly if it is over 15 mph
- They have been doing any form of combat or contact sport
- They have a head injury

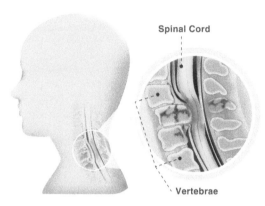

| *Spinal Injury*- Damage to spinal cord and surrounding vertebrae

If they are conscious, encourage them to remain completely still, but do not restrain them. You want to avoid them twisting.

Log-rolling someone into the recovery position

If they are unresponsive but breathing, you will need to very carefully put them into the recovery position, ideally by log-rolling.

It is rare for someone to have suffered a spinal injury, but it is vital to be cautious. It is possible to have broken your back or neck and not be aware of this until it is X-rayed. It is incredibly important to keep the spine in line and avoid them twisting. If someone has a damaged spinal column (bones) and twists, it can damage the spinal cord and result in paralysis.

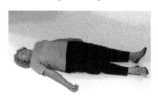
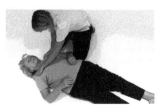

To assess their level of consciousness, first speak to them. Shout assertively and clearly, tell them who you are and ask if they are okay. If there is no response, pinch their ears or nail bed. You want to give them a sharp, painful stimulus to see if they are alive or not. If you don't get a response when you pinch one ear, pinch the other, in case they have a weakness down one side. If you get a response, you know they are alive and breathing.

If there is no response and they are breathing, (unless you have had advanced training on MILS and recognition of early airway obstruction) they need to be put into the recovery position quickly and carefully.

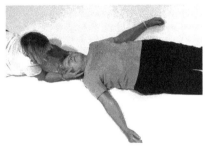

1. Support their head and neck in line with the body while you assess their level of consciousness. Do not cover their ears, as hearing is the last sense to go and the first to come back.

2. Get someone to phone for an ambulance.

3. To check if they are breathing, put your cheek above their mouth and nose; look down their body, listen to their breathing and feel their breath on your cheek.

4. Keep supporting their head and neck. Very carefully straighten their limbs and quickly prepare to log roll them into the recovery position. Check the pocket on the side that you are rolling them onto is empty.

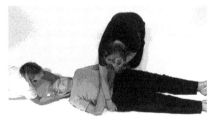

5. The second person should position themselves at the shoulders and be ready to roll the casualty towards them.

6. The third person should position themselves in the middle of the body and overlap hands to thoroughly support the casualty's body.

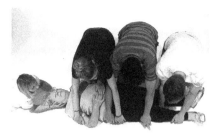

7. The fourth person supports the legs. They need to gutter the leg supporting underneath, so that when the casualty is rolled over they remain completely straight.

8. Check everyone is ready. The person holding the head should take charge. On the count of 3, everyone rolls together keeping the spine in line.

9. Check the casualty is over enough to keep the airway open and allow the contents of their stomach to drain. **Keep supporting the head. Do not let go until a paramedic takes over.** The other people should continue to support the lower part of the body. **Keep checking that they are breathing.**

If you are at all concerned about their airway put them into the recovery position immediately, keep monitoring their breathing continually.

Major crush injury – 15-minute rule

If someone is crushed by a heavy object and you are able to safely remove the object **within 15 minutes,** you should do so. If a limb has been crushed for longer than 15 minutes, or if you are unsure how long they have been trapped, leave them as they are and get the emergency services on their way immediately.

If a limb has been deprived of blood supply for longer than 15 minutes, toxins will have built up. If the blood supply is suddenly restored when the heavy object is removed, these toxins can circulate quickly and cause a cardiac arrest.

Extreme caution should be taken with all serious crush injuries – if in doubt seek medical advice immediately.

Road Traffic Accidents

Accidents on the road (both as pedestrians and in vehicles) are one of the 5 top causes of accidental death and hospital admissions in adults.

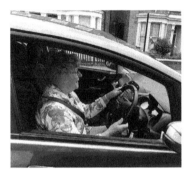

Being able to drive themselves around, is often seen as key to someone's independence. However, it is vital to ensure that someone is still safe to drive. All drivers (of any age) should be responsible for checking that their sight is good enough to drive safely, that their response times remain quick enough, and they are sufficiently alert to react to changing circumstances on the road.

Getting older can make these judgements more difficult and many people are desperate to continue to drive, when it would be prudent and safer for everyone if they didn't. We understand this predicament, having had to stop my mother driving when it became apparent that she was muddled and went to church at 11pm, oblivious of the fact it was pitch dark. The decision to stop driving is not easy and can be a major knock to an older person's confidence, undoubtedly impacting upon their sense of independence.

In most communities there are other transport options, from lift sharing, free transport, taxis and public transport and the savings in no longer running a car, can make paid options an economical alternative.

Road traffic accidents

In most EU Countries, people learn first aid as part of their driving test, but this does not happen in the UK. Accidents happen and, if involved in an accident, it is a legal requirement for all drivers to stop at the scene (only certain health professionals have a duty of care to help anyone who is injured).

There are many different types of seizure and many causes. Any head injury or stress to the brain can cause fitting; as can brain tumours, meningitis, malaria, eclampsia in pregnancy, poisoning, lack of oxygen, raised body temperature, stroke, epilepsy, drug and alcohol use and withdrawal etc.

Epilepsy

A diagnosis of epilepsy is made when someone has had at least one unprovoked seizure that cannot be attributed to any other cause.

1 in 20 people will experience some sort of a seizure during their lives. 1 in 131 are diagnosed with epilepsy.

Tonic/clonic fits and generalised seizures

What might happen

Tonic phase – they collapse to the ground as they lose consciousness. The body goes stiff and rigid and they may cry out as if in pain. This is an involuntary action as the muscles force air out of the lungs; the casualty is not in pain and is usually unaware of the noise they are making. They may begin to appear blue around their mouth and finger tips.

Clonic phase – they rigidly jerk around as the muscles alternately relax and tighten. They may make a snoring noise as the tongue flops to the back of the airway, they may be incontinent and could bite their tongue.

Post-Ictal (post-seizure) phase – once the jerking stops, they may be confused, sleepy, agitated or unresponsive (if you are worried about their airway put them in the recovery position). They may not know who they or you are, and it could take a few minutes for it to all piece back together.

Help for a generalised seizure

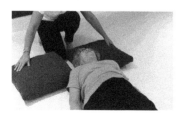

- Make sure they are safe, ease them to the ground if they are on a chair
- Protect their head without restraining them

Make a note of the time that the seizure started and of the different phases – be as detailed as you can as this is extremely useful to the medical team when investigating causes and instigating treatment. Specific information as to whether one side of the body is more affected than the other etc. can give the clinician help with their diagnosis.

- Loosen any tight clothes
- Remove any objects they could hurt themselves against
- Ask bystanders to move away to protect the casualty's dignity
- Once the seizure has stopped, check their airway and breathing
- Stay with the casualty and talk to them reassuringly throughout the seizure

Phone for an ambulance:

- If it is their first seizure
- If the seizure lasts for more than 5 minutes
- If they have another seizure straight after their first
- If they are injured
- If they are known to have seizures and this one is different in any way
- If you are worried at all
- If they are unresponsive for more than 5 minutes after the seizure

What not to do:

- **Never** put your fingers or anything in their mouth to try and prevent them biting their tongue – this will cause serious injury
- Do **not** try and move them unless they are in immediate danger
- Do **not** restrain their movements while they are fitting
- Do **not** give them anything to eat or drink until they are fully recovered
- **Never** try and "bring them round"

Early signs can be flu-like symptoms:

- Cold and shivery or hot and flushed
- Raised temperature
- Aching muscles
- Feeling very tired
- Sickness and/or diarrhoea
- Confusion

Initially blood vessels may dilate to try and attack the infection. Blood pressure drops due to the dilation of blood vessels, the heart beats faster to try and maintain blood pressure within the dilated blood vessels. Respiratory rate increases, and clotting may be affected. As sepsis progresses the body starts to go into shock. The heart struggles to maintain the necessary output and blood vessels may start to constrict to try and conserve blood to the vital organs. Eventually organs begin to fail, leading to multi-organ failure.

The exact physiology differs with individual patients.

Sepsis can be hard to recognise at first as early symptoms are similar to flu and other common illnesses. Symptoms are also similar to Meningitis.

Common signs and symptoms of meningitis and sepsis.
Symptoms can appear in any order. Some may not appear at all.

Dislike bright lights

Stiff neck

Vomiting

Severe muscle pain

Drowsy, difficult to wake

Pale, blotchy skin Spots/rash

Convulsions /seizures

Severe headache

Fever, cold hands and feet

Confusion and irritability

| For a free copy of this poster, email emma@firstaidforlife.org.uk

When to get urgent medical help:

If someone is getting worse and you are worried or if they are seriously unwell and have some of the above symptoms. **If you are sent home from the hospital or GP surgery and the casualty is getting worse, go back. Trust your instincts and tell them you are worried. Be the advocate for the casualty!**

Diabetes

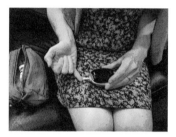

Diabetes is a condition where someone is unable to adequately regulate their blood glucose levels. The body produces the hormone insulin which helps the body burn off the sugars that are eaten. If the body has problems with insulin production, the sufferer will develop Diabetes.

Types of Diabetes

Type 1 diabetes usually develops in childhood. It occurs when the body is unable to produce any insulin. Type 1 diabetes is treated with insulin injections, or by using an insulin pump.

Type 2 diabetes is the most widespread form of the condition and tends to develop later in life, or is can be linked to obesity. Type 2 diabetes develops when the body is unable to make enough insulin, or when the insulin that is produced does not work properly (known as insulin resistance). Type 2 Diabetes is controlled by diet, exercise, oral medication, or a combination of all three, and may require insulin.

The inability to control metabolism leads to diabetics having high or low levels of glucose in their blood. First aid treatment for diabetes is more likely to be for low blood sugar levels than high. Blood sugar can drop very quickly if a diabetic has missed a meal or done additional exercise that they hadn't anticipated. High blood sugar levels usually build over a few days or weeks.

If you are looking after someone who develops weight loss, excessive urination, thirst and tiredness, these are symptoms of hyperglycaemia and they should get urgent medical attention. If they get worse and begin to get drowsy or start to lose consciousness, phone for an ambulance.

Low blood sugar/Hypoglycaemia

Hypoglycaemia is particularly dangerous as brain cells rely upon glucose as their fuel. Without sufficient glucose in the bloodstream, you lose consciousness and, without treatment, can die. Blood glucose levels can drop very quickly if someone who is diabetic has skipped a meal, done a lot of exercise, is ill, or has given themselves too much insulin.

Signs and symptoms of hypoglycaemia

- Behaving unusually

- Being aggressive

- Appearing slightly confused or drunk

- Being pale, cold, shaky and sweaty

- Shallow, rapid breathing and a fast, strong pulse

- Seizures

Treatment

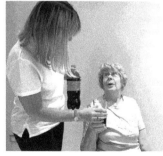

- Sit them down and give them a sugary drink or glucose sweets (not a diet drink)

- If they begin to feel better, give them more drinks and some food. Biscuits or bread will sustain their blood sugar – a jam sandwich is ideal.

- If they don't feel better within 10 minutes, or they begin to get worse, phone the emergency services. Paramedics carry Glucagon, which releases glucose from the cells.

- If they lose consciousness, but are breathing, put them in the recovery position and phone the emergency services. Keep checking they are breathing.

- If they stop breathing, start CPR

Do **not** attempt to give an unconscious casualty anything to eat or drink. **Never** give them insulin as this will further lower their blood sugar and can kill them.

Warning: Even if someone appears to have recovered, ensure they receive medical advice as soon as possible. This is particularly important at night, as insulin is still active in the bloodstream while you are sleeping. This means blood sugar levels will therefore drop again, so they could drift from sleeping to unconsciousness.

After the emergency – THE AFTERMATH

What happens after an accident is important too. It is vital that all efforts are made to ensure no further incidents occur because of this one.

NB: If it is possible that there may need to be a criminal investigation or police involvement following the incident, then always check with them first before moving or cleaning anything.

1. Clear up. Ensure you remove/clean up any body fluids that could represent a hazard safely and appropriately. Hygienically dispose of contaminated items in a yellow incinerator bag or sanitary bin. Remove faulty equipment or anything else that could pose a danger to others.

2. Ensure that appropriate paperwork and accident forms are completed.

3. Restock anything that has been used from a first aid kit.

4. Ensure that everyone is okay afterwards – dealing with a medical emergency can be extremely stressful and some people need professional help and counselling following such an episode.

5. It is perfectly normal to feel any of the following after an accident:
- Elation/an adrenaline buzz
- Anger
- Confusion
- Flashbacks and bad dreams
- Depression

Part 4

Useful information

What to put in your first aid kit

First aid kits need to be well-stocked and easily accessible. They should be well organised; ideally in a bag with compartments to allow you to grab what you need as quickly as possible. It is most important that the kits contents are good quality. Cheap kits are often not of sufficient quality.

Your kit should contain a first aid book or instructions, and contents to treat major and minor bleeding, burns, breaks and sprains. The kit should not contain medication. First aid kits for a car should be in soft padded cases or secured within the car.

Essential contents

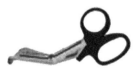

Tough cut scissors – strong enough to cut through clothes

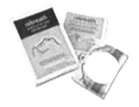

A face shield - to protect yourself when doing mouth-to-mouth resuscitation

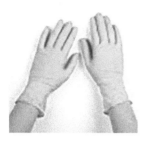

Gloves – non-sterile to protect you, and sterile for treating someone with deep wounds or burns

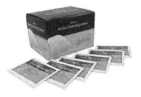

Sterile medical wipes - to clean wounds

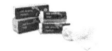

Wound dressings - of various sizes

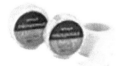

Micropore tape - to secure dressings and tape fingers and toes, also useful for labelling things

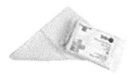

A couple of calico triangular bandages - ensure they are calico, not a cheap version made of paper as these are some of the most useful things in your kit. They are sterile, non-fluffy material, useful for stopping bleeding, for slings and support bandages, and far easier than a dressing to secure on head, knee and elbow wounds.

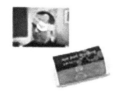
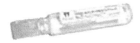

Eye dressings

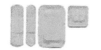

Sterile saline vial – for irrigating a wound or washing grit from an eye

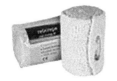

Crepe bandage – for supporting a sprain or strain

Plasters – for short-term covering of a minor wound (do not use for more than an hour or so as wounds can become soggy)

Additional useful contents

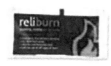

Burn gel or a burns dressing – to apply to a burn after cooling

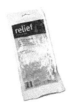

Instant ice pack – at home you can use a bag of frozen peas, but ensure it is wrapped in a cloth, otherwise it can cause ice burns

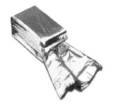

A foil blanket - to keep casualties warm, crucially important in helping to prevent them going into shock.

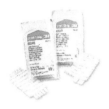

Steri-strips - to help close gaping wounds

Sterile tweezers – for removing small splinters

Accident forms

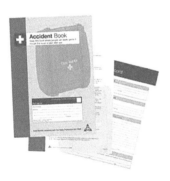

A minor injury can lead to a major problem, so all injuries should be recorded either on a formal accident form if you are a business or formal carer, or in a designated book if you are a home carer.

Accident books will be inspected and may be able to show trends and patterns of injuries which can lead to improvements in Health and Safety.

Proper accident recording can be vital written defence should there ever be a legal challenge concerning the accident, injury or treatment given.

An accident book is a legal document. Things recorded at the time of an accident are usually considered to be more reliable evidence than those recalled from memory.

An accident record should be completed as soon as possible after the incident. The entire report should be completed in one go, in the same ballpoint or non-erasable pen.

The report should contain the following information:

- The full name of the casualty
- The casualty's occupation
- The date, time and location of the incident
- What happened, in as much detail as possible
- What injuries were sustained
- Treatment given
- Medical help sought (if any)
- Witnesses – names and contact details
- Layout of area – including a sketch if possible
- Further action required
- The name, address, occupation and signature of the person completing the report

It is good practice to state whether someone has refused medical intervention and their reasons for this. Seek medical advice if you are unsure whether they are fully conscious and in a suitable state of mind to be able to make this decision.

Accident books can be bought from many sources and are widely available online through the HSE.

The book needs to comply with the Data Protection Act and therefore personal records need to be removed and stored securely, and a member of staff designated to be responsible for the safekeeping of accident records within a lockable cabinet.

The person who has had the accident or their legal guardian is entitled to a copy of the report. This should be copied prior to filing and they should keep a record of the accident report number.

Reporting of Accidents and Incidents at Work: RIDDOR 1995 regulations

Reporting of Injuries, Diseases and Dangerous Occurrences Regulations 1995.

It is the responsibility of the Employer or person in charge of the premises to report the following occurrences directly to the Health and Safety Executive:

The following should be reported immediately:

- Death
- Major injuries
- Dangerous occurrences
- An incident that results in someone taking time off work (or being unable to perform full duties) for more than 3 days. This needs to be reported within 10 days.
- Notifiable diseases. These should be reported as soon as possible.

Part 5

RESOURCES

Risk Assessment for Care Workers

The principal objective of home care is the provision of support to enable people to be cared for in their own home for as long as possible, or to enable them to return to their own home from hospital or other accommodation. Home care workers assist people at home, allowing them to stay in their homes, rather than use residential, long-term, or nursing care institutions. Care workers visit users to help with daily tasks, and assist in their physical personal needs and in the follow-up of medical plans.

The following risk assessment has been drawn up by the European Agency for Safety and Health at Work. Part A is a risk assessment and part B is suggested preventative measures to aid safer working.

Risk assessment checklist for Home care workers

The general checklist is a tool to help identify hazards in the carer's workplace.

Part A: Does the hazard exist at the workplace?

YES – if you have ticked at least one answer in a field marked with ☐

Please note that the list below does not cover all the possible cases in which there are hazards.

QUESTION	YES	NO
1. DRIVING TO THE PATIENT'S HOME		
1.1 Is the client expecting the carer?	☐	☐
1.2 Is the home in a high crime area or an isolated location?	☐	☐
2. DANGEROUS BEHAVIOUR OF PERSONS OUTSIDE THE HOME		
2.1 Is the home in a high crime area or an isolated location?	☐	☐
2.2 Does the carer travel alone?	☐	☐
3. THE PHYSICAL ENVIRONMENT OUTSIDE THE HOME		
3.1 Are the surfaces sometimes slippery, e.g. when wet, muddy or dusty?	☐	☐
3.2 Does the ground have uneven areas, loose covering, holes, spills etc.?	☐	☐
3.3 Are there thresholds or other changes of level on outside surfaces?	☐	☐
3.4 Is the lighting of surfaces and access routes inadequate?	☐	☐
3.5 Are animals present?	☐	☐
4. THE PHYSICAL ENVIRONMENT INSIDE THE HOME Fire – explosion		
4.1 Are appropriate fire precautions in place (smoke detectors, extinguishers, ...)? (where relevant)	☐	☐
4.2 Is there any damaged insulation on wires (e.g. kinks or exposed wires)?	☐	☐
4.3 Is there any damage to electrical equipment housing, or housing not present?	☐	☐
4.4 Are there any damaged plugs or sockets?	☐	☐

4.5 Are there any overloaded electrical sockets? ☐ ☐

4.6 Are oxidising or flammable substances, such as paint, finishes, adhesives and solvents used? ☐ ☐

4.7 Are oxygen cylinders safely stored in a proper location? ☐ ☐

4.8 Is propane, butane or natural gas in use in the client's home? ☐ ☐

Lighting

4.9 Is lighting adequate to perform tasks efficiently, accurately and safely? ☐ ☐

4.10 Is the lighting of circulation areas, corridors, stairs, rooms, etc., adequate to move safely and to notice any obstacle (holes in the ground, objects lying on the ground, steps, slippery surfaces or spills, etc.)? ☐ ☐

Animals

4.11 Are animals present? ☐ ☐

Floor and stairs

4.12 Do the floors have uneven areas, loose coverings, holes, spills, etc.? ☐ ☐

4.13 Are the floors sometimes slippery, e.g. when they are wet due to cleaning or spilling of liquids, or dusty due to construction work? ☐ ☐

4.14 Are there thresholds or other changes of level on the floors? ☐ ☐

4.15 Are the floors kept tidy? ☐ ☐

4.16 Are there cables on the floor? ☐ ☐

4.17 Are there any obstructions and objects (excluding those which cannot be removed) left lying around in the work area? ☐ ☐

4.18 Could the carer fall or slip due to unsuitable footwear? ☐ ☐

4.19 Are client's home stairs in poor condition or cluttered? ☐ ☐

5. ACTIVITIES OF DAILY LIVING General

5.1 Is training required to safely assist clients in the activities of daily living? ☐ ☐

5.2 Client care activities, especially client handling activities, can put the carer at high risk. Do the activities of daily living include: transferring or repositioning, dressing and bathing clients? ☐ ☐

5.3 Do the activities of transferring or repositioning the client involve manual handling, reaching, bending or twisting? ☐ ☐

5.4 Are there risks of acute injuries? (back pain from lifting a client, shoulder pain by trying to stop a client from falling, moving heavy objects such as furniture) ☐ ☐

5.5 Are there risks of chronic injuries? (High repetition activities with excessive force, awkward posture, static load or direct pressure on the tissues) ☐ ☐

5.6 Is more than one person needed to assist with tasks like bathing, repositioning and transferring? ☐ ☐

Transferring and repositioning

5.7 Does the client resist being moved? ☐ ☐

5.8 Does the carer need further information about adequate transferring and repositioning techniques? ☐ ☐

Dressing

5.9 Does the activity of dressing the client involve reaching and excessive bending or the adoption of an awkward posture? ☐ ☐

5.10 During dressing does one of the client's limbs (arm or leg) have to be supported for a long time or require the exertion of a high force? ☐ ☐

5.11 Does the carer need further information about
adequate dressing technique? ☐ ☐

Bathing

5.12 When bathing a client does this require the
adoption of an awkward or static posture, high
forces or high contact stress (on knees from
kneeling or upper chest from leaning against
the bath)? ☐ ☐

5.13 Does the carer need further information about
adequate bathing technique? ☐ ☐

Assistive devices

5.14 Are assistive devices required to safely meet the
demands of the activities of daily living? ☐ ☐

5.15 Is training required to work with assistive
devices? ☐ ☐

6. DOMESTIC DUTIES

6.1 Housekeeping activities can put the carer at
high risk. Do the activities include: making
beds, cleaning, doing laundry and cooking? ☐ ☐

6.2 Do the activities of bed making and tucking in
sheets require bending over at the waist and
reaching forward or gripping sheets and bed
covers using a pinch grip (which increases the
effort required)? ☐ ☐

6.3 Does the activity of cleaning the floors, the
toilet or the bath involve bending over or
kneeling? ☐ ☐

6.4 Does the activity of cleaning overhead require
reaching overhead for a long time? ☐ ☐

6.5 Does scrubbing with force require bending
or reaching? ☐ ☐

6.6 Do domestic activities require kneeling on hard
surfaces which can put pressure on the knees? ☐ ☐

6.7 Does loading or unloading laundry from washers and dryers require repeated bending forward while twisting? □ □

6.8 Does lifting dry laundry require using a pinch grip (which can increase the forces of the small muscles in the hand and forearm)? □ □

6.9 Is lifting wet laundry part of the domestic duties? □ □

6.10 Does food preparation and cooking involve the use of blunt knives which can increase the force required to cut food? □ □

6.11 Is the work surface height appropriate for preparing and cooking food? (For example if it is too low it can require bending over and putting stress on the back, whilst too high can require the use of awkward wrist and shoulder postures). □ □

6.12 Are cleaning products used in the client's home as they can put the carer at risk of exposure to chemicals? □ □

7. THE PATIENT'S HEALTH CONDITION (INFECTIOUS CONDITIONS)

Blood-borne diseases

7.1 Does the client have a blood-borne disease (e.g. HIV/AIDS or Hepatitis B/C)? □ □

7.2 Does the client have a wound, active bleeding or wound drainage? □ □

7.3 Does the client require assistance with bowel or bladder elimination? □ □

7.4 Can infected blood or body fluids come into contact with the tissue lining of the carer's eyes, nose, or mouth? □ □

7.5 Can infected blood or body fluids come into contact with a cut in the skin? □ □

7.6 Can the care worker be accidentally pricked with a needle or a sharp (lancet, for example) that is contaminated with infected blood? ☐ ☐

7.7 Can the carer prevent exposure to blood-borne diseases? ☐ ☐

7.8 Does the carer know what to do in the case of unprotected contact with potentially infected blood or body fluids? ☐ ☐

Airborne diseases

7.9 Does the client have an airborne disease (e.g. flu, tuberculosis, measles, chicken pox or influenza)? ☐ ☐

7.10 Could the care worker touch a person or object (e.g., table, doorknob, or telephone) contaminated with the disease, and then touch their own eyes, nose, or mouth? ☐ ☐

7.11 Could the care worker breathe in the very small airborne drops of saliva or mucus produced when an infected person coughs, sneezes or speaks very close to them? ☐ ☐

7.12 Does the carer know what to do to prevent exposure to airborne diseases? ☐ ☐

Contact diseases

7.13 Does the client have an infectious disease that can be spread by contact (e.g. herpes, MRSA, scabies, rubella, mumps or ringworm)? ☐ ☐

7.14 Could the care worker touch a person or object (e.g. table, doorknob, telephone) contaminated with the disease, and then touch their own eyes, nose, or mouth? ☐ ☐

7.15 Does the carer know what to do to prevent exposure to contactdiseases? ☐ ☐

8. PSYCHOSOCIAL ISSUES

Client behaviour including violence

8.1 Does the client demonstrate or have a history of behaviour, such as verbal attacks, threats of physical attack or actual physical attacks? ☐ ☐

8.2 Does the client have a mental illness? (e.g. a mental health diagnosis, depression, paranoia, confusion, agitation?) ☐ ☐

8.3 Are there any recognised events or conditions that bring about violent or aggressive behaviour in the patient? ☐ ☐

8.4 Are there significant changes in the client's mood? ☐ ☐

8.5 Does the carer have difficulty in communicating with the client? ☐ ☐

Family members and visitors

8.6 Do family members and/or visitors have a history of violent behaviour? ☐ ☐

8.7 Do family members often become argumentative? ☐ ☐

8.8 Are there any unexpected client visitors? ☐ ☐

8.9 Does the carer feel a lack of consideration from the family members? ☐ ☐

Time pressure

8.10 Does the carer feel that the time available is not enough to assist the client? ☐ ☐

9. EMERGENCIES

9.1 Does an emergency action plan exist for the client's home? ☐ ☐

9.2 Does the carer have contact phone numbers in the case of an emergency? ☐ ☐

9.3 Does the carer know the fastest evacuation route in the case of an emergency? ☐ ☐

10. INFORMATION AND TRAINING

10.1 Does the carer know about the hazards they are exposed to? ☐ ☐

10.2 Does the carer know how they may be affected by the hazards they are exposed to? ☐ ☐

10.3 Did the carer receive appropriate instructions regarding health and safety risks? ☐ ☐

10.4 Did the carer receive adequate safety and health training? ☐ ☐

11. HEALTH SURVEILLANCE

11.1 Did the carer receive health surveillance appropriate to the health and safety risks they incur at work? ☐ ☐

The proposed solutions presented in Part B are examples of preventive measures that can be taken to reduce risks. The solutions correspond directly to the questions in Part A.

Part B: Examples of preventive measures that can reduce risk

QUESTION N°.	EXAMPLES OF PREVENTIVE MEASURES
	1. DRIVING TO THE PATIENT'S HOME
1.1	Informing the client before travelling; finding out who should be in the home.
1.2	Carrying an extra set of car keys, a torch, a mobile phone and possibly a personal alarm when visiting a client; planning the safest route to the client's home; keeping the car well maintained; taking precautions in the event of a car breakdown.

2. THE DANGEROUS BEHAVIOUR OF PERSONS OUTSIDE THE HOME

2.1   Don't leave personal items visible in the car; when it is dark, park your car in a open spot near a streetlight.

2.2   When travelling and working alone, the risk of exposure to violent behaviour can be reduced by: sticking to busy roads and streets, locking the car while driving, avoiding bus stops that are poorly lit or where there are few people, walking directly to the nearest place of business – without running or looking back – if you feel you are being followed.

3. THE PHYSICAL ENVIRONMENT OUTSIDE THE HOME

3.1   If necessary, treating slippery surfaces chemically, using appropriate cleaning methods.

3.2   Selecting flooring and ground surfaces carefully, especially if likely to become wet or dusty.

3.3   Ensuring ground surfaces and access routes are checked regularly.

3.4   Ensuring adequate lighting of surfaces and access routes; reporting broken light bulbs outside the home.

3.5   Ensuring aggressive pets are leashed or locked up in a separate room before leaving the car or entering a home.

4. THE PHYSICAL ENVIRONMENT INSIDE THE HOME

Fire – explosion

4.1   Ensuring that smoke detectors are checked regularly (where relevant).

4.1   Ensuring appropriate choice of fire extinguishers, appropriate location, checking and regular servicing (where relevant).

4.2   Carrying out a visual check for defects; using only equipment
4.3   with the EC mark; ensuring that defects are repaired by an
4.4   electrical expert.

4.5   Limiting the number of appliances connected to the same socket.

4.6   Ensuring the appropriate storage of combustible or flammable substances.

4.7   Oxygen is a fire hazard; keeping all sources of flame away from oxygen cylinders; storing oxygen cylinders in a rack, or chained to the wall, in a well-ventilated area.

4.8   Never use a gas appliance if unsure whether it is working properly. Ensuring that a gas safety check is done. If smelling gas, or suspecting there is a gas escape, immediately open all doors and windows and shut off the gas supply at the meter control valve. If gas continues to escape call the Gas Emergency Number. In the case of a suspected carbon monoxide leakage, unless you are able to identify the specific appliance at fault, consult a qualified installer to investigate and make repairs.[12]

Lighting

4.9   Lighting intensity and uniformity must be adequate to the work; increasing the wattage of a bulb if more lighting is
4.10   needed; using additional local or localised lighting where high levels of lighting are required.

Animals

4.11   Ensuring that aggressive pets are leashed or locked in a separate room before leaving the car or entering the home.

4.12	Selecting flooring carefully, especially if it is likely to become wet or dusty; anti-slip and easy-to-clean surfaces are preferable.
4.13	

4.14	Ensuring floor is checked regularly.

4.15	Repairing holes and cracks, worn carpets or rugs, etc.; keeping floors clear.

4.16	Positioning equipment to avoid cables crossing a working area; using cable covers to fix them securely to surfaces.

4.17	Removing holes, cracks, worn carpets or rugs, etc.; keeping floors clear.

4.18	Using suitable footwear (comfortable and anti-slip).

4.19	Keeping stairs free of clutter; they must have handrails and be well lit.

5. ACTIVITIES OF DAILY LIVING

5.1	The employer must ensure that proper health and safety information, instruction and training for work activities are provided to care workers.

5.2	Performing only those tasks for which training has been provided.

5.3	Understanding the risks of musculoskeletal disorders (MSDs) and working safely within one's physical capabilities.

5.4	Never try to hold a client in a standing position; never try to stop a client from falling, but rather control the client's fall to the floor as trained; using mechanical aids to move heavy objects; using equipment such as portable lifts whenever possible; working in pairs or teams to lighten the load (when possible).

5.5   Avoiding pinch grips, using a power grip instead of a pinch grip; reducing awkward shoulder, wrist or trunk postures; taking short breaks to rest the lower back, neck, shoulders or wrists; alternating static with dynamic postures and activities.

5.6   Informing employers that more than one person is needed; working in pairs or teams to lighten the load (when possible).

Transferring and repositioning

5.7   Checking for hazards and assessing the risks when transferring or repositioning a client.

5.8   Ensuring adequate training and technique for transferring or repositioning clients:

- Using transfer assist devices such as transfer belts or lowfriction slide sheets;

- Accessing a position close to the client by removing obstacles from around bed and chair; avoiding the client holding on to the carer;

- Working in pairs or teams to lighten the load (when possible);

- Using proper techniques: during a transfer or repositioning task, shift the body weight using legs. Don't pull with the arms or back;

- Ensuring a strong base of support, by keeping the feet a shoulders-width apart, by positioning one foot forward and one foot back, by bending the knees and by keeping the back straight;

- Avoiding holding a client in a standing position;

- Controlling the client's fall to the floor as trained; avoiding trying to stop a client from falling;

- Using a strong power grip and avoiding pinch grips.

5.9   Asking the client to assist as much as possible; using a proper technique for dressing clients.

5.10   Using equipment such as portable lifts whenever possible.

5.11   Ensuring adequate technique for dressing clients:

- Using proper techniques. When helping the client move, keep the body upright and shift the body weight using the legs;

- Starting with the client's weaker side when putting on clothes;

- Helping the client to lean forward when putting on shirts; this will relax the client's arms;

- Trying to complete several tasks at the same time. For example: rolling the client to a place on an incontinence pad, pulling on a pant leg, and adjusting a lift sling;

- Sitting on a stool when helping seated clients to put on their socks and shoes;

- Ensuring that the client is as close to the side of the bed as possible;

- Accessing a position close to the client by removing obstacles from around bed and chair;

- Sitting on the bed, or putting one knee up on it, to bring the carer closer to the client;

- Placing a client's lower legs on a small stool or other elevated surface to lift their thighs off the bed;

- Clothing can be adapted to make dressing clients easier. For example, adaptive clothing is roomier than normal clothing, has elasticised waistbands, and uses oversized buttons, snap fasteners or Velcro fastenings.

Bathing

5.12   Asking the client to assist as much as possible; using a propertechnique for bathing clients.

5.13   Ensuring adequate technique for bathing clients:

- Planning the bathing process. Assemble everything needed, and position all equipment. In small bathrooms, pulling the wheelchair from the front to avoid climbing around it;

- Seating clients on a transfer bench or shower stool before helping them into the bath, and lather the far side of their bodies. Place the client's feet on a stool or the edge of the bath and lather them;

- Sitting on a stool, the side of the bath or on the toilet seat (if it's closer) will keep the carer's back more upright and reduce the need to reach and bend;

- Using grab bars (if available) with one hand to support carer's upper body;

- Taking short breaks to rest the carer's lower back (e.g. standing up straight and arching the back slightly backwards);

- When bathing a client in bed trying not to twist, bend, or reach for water. Place the water basins on a stool or table at a comfortable height and close to where the carer is working.

Assistive devices

5.14   Different assistive devices may be used in the activities of daily living. Lifting equipment, transfer benches, sliding boards, lowfriction slide sheets or posts may be required in helping to get the client in and out of bed or to help the client when walking; a wheelchair may be required to transfer the client between different locations; a shower chair or a transfer bench for the bathroom may be required to assist clients during bathing; a small stool or other elevated surface may be required to lift a client's thighs off the bed.

- Using appropriate personal protective equipment (including gloves, gown, goggles, face shield, and respirator) as trained;

- Wearing gloves, gowns and mask, when in contact with contaminated objects;

- Ensure that infectious clients wear surgical masks;

- Understanding the risk assessment results from the carer's manager, and following the recommended safe work procedures.

Contact diseases

7.13   Ensuring that the carer receives the training to interact with clients with contact diseases. Ensuring that the carer has available basic protective equipment such as disposable gloves, gowns and disinfecting equipment.

7.14   If the carer is exposed to contact diseases (e.g., herpes, MRSA, scabies, rubella, mumps or ringworm), particular precautions must be taken to assure that the carer will not be contaminated by the disease.

7.15   Adequate actions and provisions to protect carers from airborne diseases include[9]:

- Having the appropriate vaccinations and booster shots;

- Trying not to touch the eyes, face or mouth during work;

- Washing the hands frequently using proper hand washing procedure;

- Using appropriate personal protective equipment (including gloves and gown) as trained;

- Not washing and re - using gloves;

- Understanding the risk assessment results from the carer's manager, and following the recommended safe work

8. PSYCHOSOCIAL ISSUES

Client behavior including violence

8.1　The carer may leave the home when feeling threatened; use specific techniques to calm the family members and visitors, as trained; refrain from arguing or raising the voice; try to maintain a safe distance from the client.

8.2　Being aware of any mental health diagnoses.

8.3　Being aware of specific triggers, and ways to minimise violent behaviour; being informed if the client has a history of violent behaviour.

8.4　When arriving at the client's home, assess the client's mood before starting work.

8.5　Contact carer manager or patient family members to find different ways to communicate with the client.

Family members and visitors

8.6　Being informed of violent behaviour from the client's family.

8.7　The carer may leave the home when feeling threatened; using specific techniques to calm the family members and visitors, as trained

8.8　The carer may ask the client to ask an unexpected visitor to leave before entering or before providing care.

8.9　Contacting carer manager; using specific techniques to increase the trust of the family members in the carer's job; the carer may leave the home when feeling threatened.

Time pressure

8.10　Contacting the carer's manager.

9. EMERGENCIES

9.1　An emergency action plan must be prepared for the client's home:

9.2　　• Identifying home evacuation procedures;

9.3　　• Identifying the fastest way for an evacuation (escape routes);

Drug interactions and hospitalisation in older patients

(www.nejm.org/doi/full/10.1056/NEJMsa1103053#t=abstract)

www.betterhealthwhileaging.net/

Safety resources:

Institute of Home Safety (national)

The London Home and Water Safety Council

Royal Society for the Prevention of Accidents RoSPA

www.riddor.gov.uk

Health and Safety Executive latest guidance on first aid training (http://www.hse.gov.uk/firstaid/first-aid-training.htm http://www.hse.gov.uk/pubns/priced/l74.pdf)

www.hse.gov.uk/firstaid/legislation.htm#duties

Age UK
Care UK
www.firstaidforlife.org.uk/first-aid-shop/

www.nhs.uk/Livewell/healthy-bones/Pages/falls-risk-assessment-tool.aspx

Resources for medical conditions:

The Resuscitation Council guidelines (www.resus.org.uk/)

ERC guidelines - (https://www.erc.edu/)

St John and the Red Cross 10th Edition

www.asthma.org.uk/

Anaphylaxis Trust

www.youtube.com/watch?v=CjgbwmQy2r8

How to Use a Jext

www.youtube.com/watch?v=pgvnt8YA7r8

How to Use an Epipen

Poisons database (www.npis.org/toxbase.html)

Headway brain injury (www.headway.org.uk/)

Epilepsy: www.epilepsy.org.uk/info/seizures/febrile-convulsions

Great Ormond Street Hospital advice on febrile convulsions (www.gosh.nhs.uk/parents-and-visitors/)

Sepsis Trust (sepsistrust.org/info-for-the-public/)

www.diabetes.org.uk/

I do hope this information has been useful to you.

There is no better way to learn first aid than joining one of our award-winning practical or online first aid courses.

Visit www.firstaidforlife.org.uk and www.onlinefirstaid.com for more information and loads of free resources. You can also sign up to receive updates.

Learn pet first aid with us at www.firstaidforpets.net.

For further information or to ask any questions, email emma@firstaidforlife.org.uk

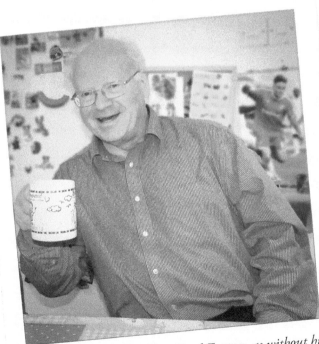

In special memory of Raymond Fenton, as without his continuing belief, practical support and ongoing enthusiasm, First Aid for Life might never have existed!

Lightning Source UK Ltd.
Milton Keynes UK
UKHW02f0237090218
317626UK00009B/56/P